Reach for Your Rainbow

A Gentle Fitness Guide

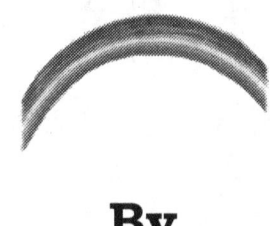

By

Brenda L. Rogers

This book is a work of non-fiction. Names and places have been changed to protect the privacy of all individuals. The events and situations are true.

First published by AuthorHouse 04/27/04

ISBN: 1-4184-5512-1 (e-book)
ISBN: 1-4184-5511-3 (Paperback)

Library of Congress Control Number: 2003090386

This book is printed on acid free paper.

Printed in the United States of America
Bloomington, IN

Edited by Todd Rogers
Photography by Blake Moulin
Design by M-M Stratton
Art by Brenda L. Rogers

Acknowledgments

This work evolved as a natural outpouring of love, interest, and support from my friends and family. Thanks especially to my son, Todd, whose tireless efforts made this book possible.

Special thanks to my ageless mother, Ruth, who gave me the freedom to pursue dance while she sat for my children.   And to my Dad, Harry, who paid for the lessons, and still cheers for me at every performance. My parents are my role models on "youthing" - keeping fit mentally, emotionally, and physically.

Thanks to Sonia Shaw, my first jazz dance instructor, who hired and empowered me as a teaching assistant soon after I rejoined her classes in my thirties.

A salute to my modern dance teachers who introduced me to the creative expression of unobstructed movement.

Gratitude to Dr. Paul Rosenberg who gave me the opportunity to explore healing with those in recovery.

To my dear friend, mentor, and teacher, Dr. Jaquelyn McCandless who inspired me to transcend my "young mother" self-image and to "reach for my rainbow."

And deepest gratitude to God who gave me my creative nature.

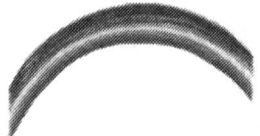

Dedication

To my parents who have shown me that love is the secret of longevity.

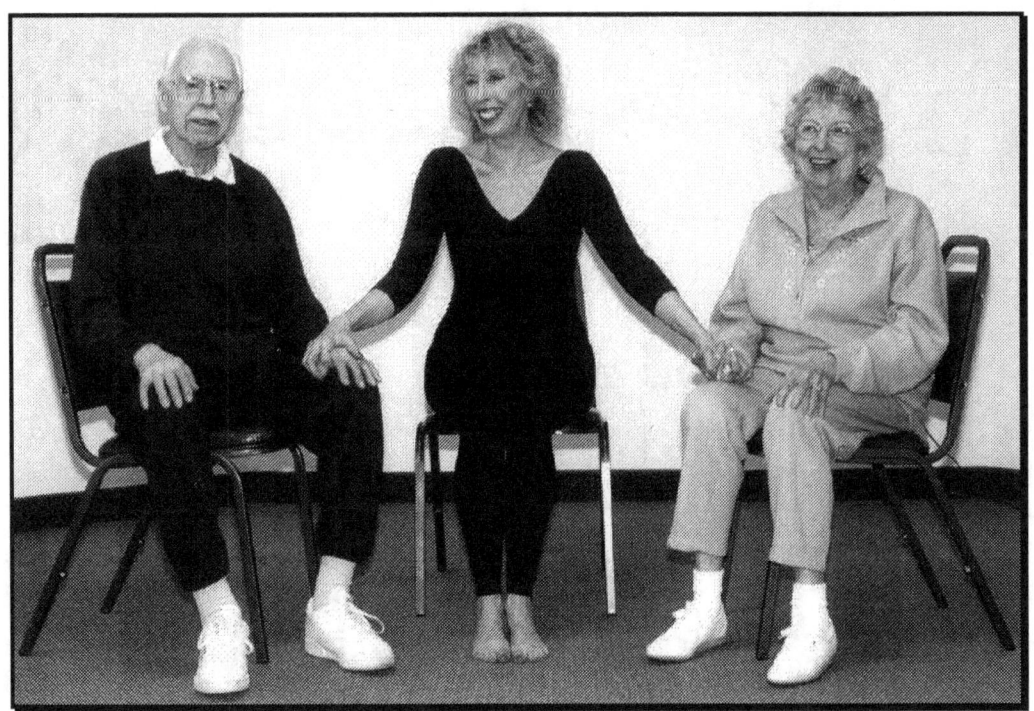

Photograph by Jeanne Adams

And to my friends, clients, students, and patients with whom I have shared this wonderful journey.

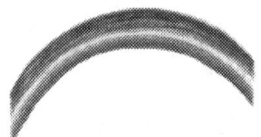

Contents

Forward

In *Reach for Your Rainbow, A Gentle Fitness Guide*, Brenda L. Rogers makes a valuable contribution to the expanding vision of healthy "elderhood" through exercise. It is well known that exercising enhances overall health. Many exercise to burn off fat and strengthen muscles to improve appearance. Health benefits of regular exercise also include strengthening the immune system, correcting poor posture, reducing stress, alleviating back pain, lifting depression, aiding digestion, increasing energy and self-confidence, and decreasing injuries.

Research shows that certain chronic diseases, such as diabetes, arthritis, and hypertension can be reduced by regular exercise. You do not feel old when you feel stronger and alive in your body. Brenda inspires us, through photos and simple explanations, to move, bend, stretch - in short, to feel good.

These 'gentle' exercises have been carefully, thoughtfully and lovingly created to help relieve aches, pains, and stiffness. Brenda engenders respect and appreciation for your body in her exercises. For the first time in years you may actually enjoy and love your body. Her work supports the body's own healing powers. You are encouraged to take charge of your health and support your body's natural inclination toward wholeness.

Recent advances in medicine, nutritional awareness, and programs like *Reach for Your Rainbow, A Gentle Fitness Guide*, are making our later years healthier and more productive. Brenda L. Rogers clearly knows and teaches that the best exercises are those you enjoy. It is much easier to stay with something that is fun to do. *Reach For Your Rainbow, A Gentle Fitness Guide* is a very welcome addition to our increasing awareness of the creative aging process. Who says we can't keep up with our youth? We will live happier, healthier and longer.

Jaquelyn McCandless, M.D., Certified by the American Board of Psychiatry and Neurology, Anti-Aging Specialist and Author of "Children With Starving Brains: A Medical Treatment Guide for Autism Spectrum Disorder."

Introduction

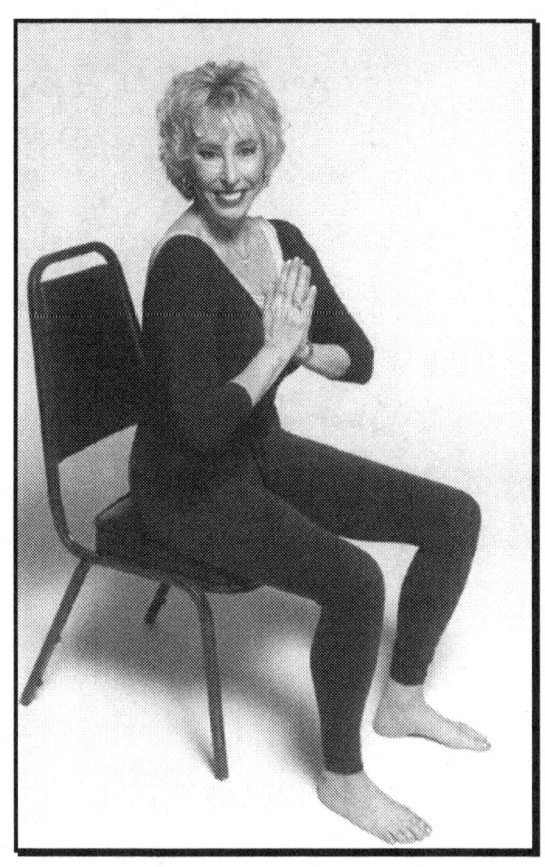

Welcome to *Reach for Your Rainbow, A Gentle Fitness Guide.*

I have always believed that simple, easy-to-perform exercises are most likely to be practiced by the greatest number of people. The following pages demonstrate many of these effective movements. This workbook is intended for everyone - regardless of age, gender, or physical condition.

Reach for Your Rainbow, A Gentle Fitness Guide is a collection of fun exercises that are geared to stimulate, elevate, and integrate both mind and body.

I hope you enjoy these exercises as much as I enjoyed developing them and performing them over the years.

Love, Joy and Peace,

Brenda

Exercises

The exercises on the following pages are titled and represented by photographs that demonstrate the basic movements. I used large print, and in some editions, a spiral binding, to create a workbook which could be placed on the floor and still remain readable to the student seated or in a standing position.

The chapter headings suggest that you work on each major area of the body in series, starting from the top – "Neck and Shoulders," "Shoulders and Upper Back," "Arms and Upper Back," and so on, down to the lower extremities. Although this order can be construed as a good working order for the student, it is equally for the sake of a reference and organization.

It is not necessary to perform every exercise in one session or in any particular order. Rather, a regimen of varying the exercises can be most effective, beneficial, and fun!

Each exercise is divided into distinct, easy-to-digest units, denoted by a representative graphic so as to, again, be highly visible and easily read during the course of this program.

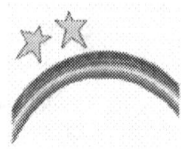 One, two, three, or four stars indicate the level of difficulty for each exercise in what I call the "Rainbow Rating Level." One star is the easiest for the beginner while four stars can be more challenging.

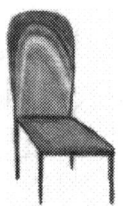 The "Rainbow Chair" marks the starting position or beginning stance for each exercise.

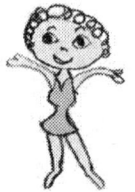 The "Leotard Lady" describes each movement in detail.

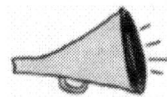 The "Bullhorn" instructs us on repetitions and the manner in which we should practice the movements.

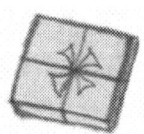 Students are always presented with a little "Gift" in all my classes. Here, I offer friendly encouragement and loving support.

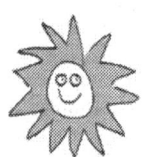 Finally, the "Sun" shines brightly on each exercise. I always use affirmations <u>to be said out loud</u> and as frequently as possible for best results.

At first, some exercises may be more strenuous than others, so <u>take your time</u>. Breathe naturally during the exercises. Read through the instructions for each exercise for a complete understanding before performing them and remember to practice your best posture - seated or standing - in an upright position. Keep in mind the following tips while performing each exercise:

- Keep your buttocks and stomach tight, shoulders down, and chest up - avoid leaning back or slouching.

- Place your feet naturally distancing them from each other.

- Plant your feet firmly and evenly on the ground to evenly distribute your weight.

- Wear loose, comfortable clothing.

- Use a sturdy, comfortable chair.

- Finally, it is foremost that you <u>listen to your body</u>.

Do not overdo it. Stay focused and centered during each activity. If you feel faint, dizzy, fatigued, or in the least bit uncomfortable, stop! Though the following "low-impact" exercises are designed to benefit in the gentlest manner, remember to always consult your physician before embarking on any physical fitness program.

After working your way up to practicing each and every exercise, I can assure you that you will be feeling better, more flexible and well on your way to reaching your rainbow!

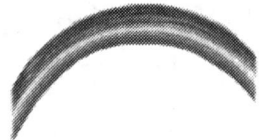

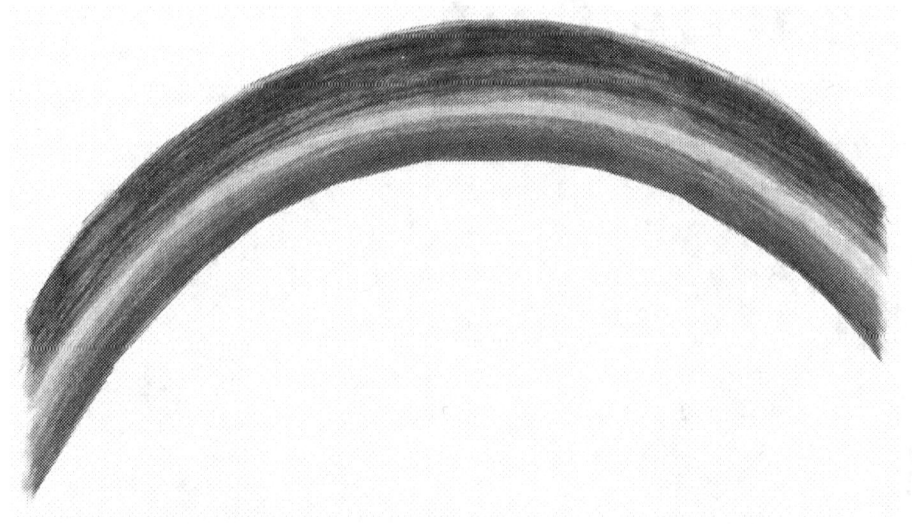

Breathing

Breathe In
Breathe Out

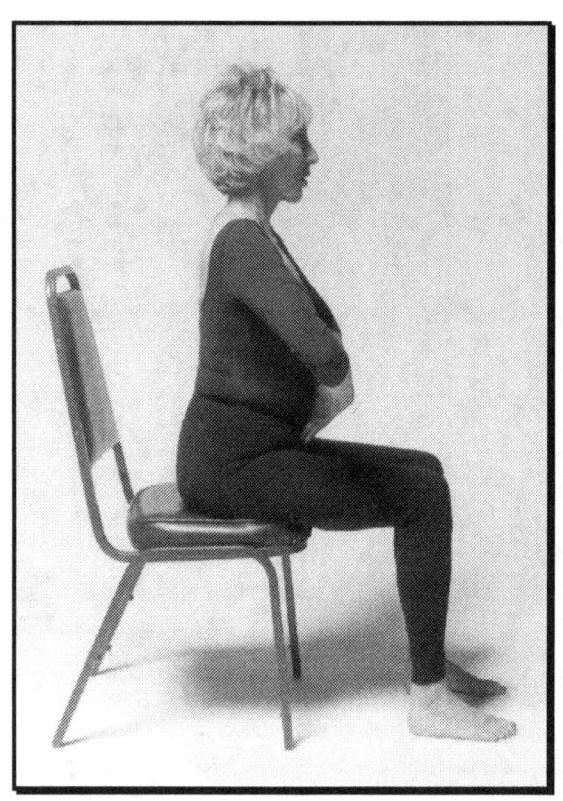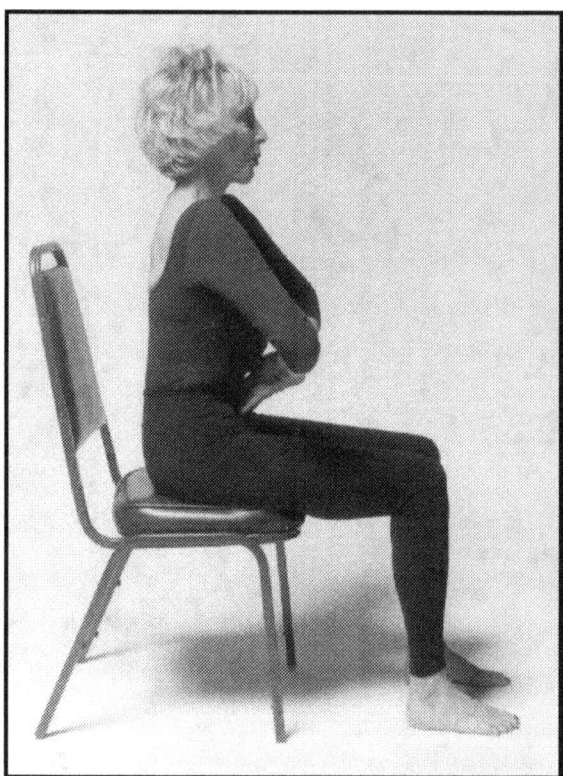

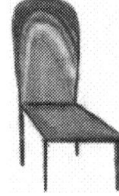 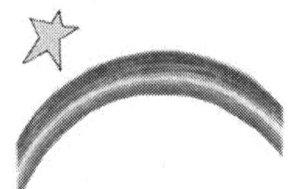 Sit tall in chair, shoulders down, chest up.

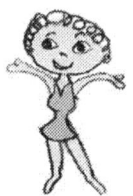 Place hands on stomach.

Inhale deeply.

Feel the mid-section expand.

Exhale and empty lungs.

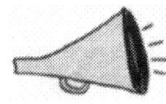 Repeat this deep breathing – in and out.

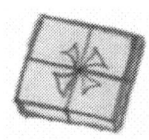 Way to go!

"The universe fills me with good.
I let go of the past."

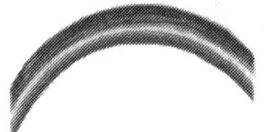

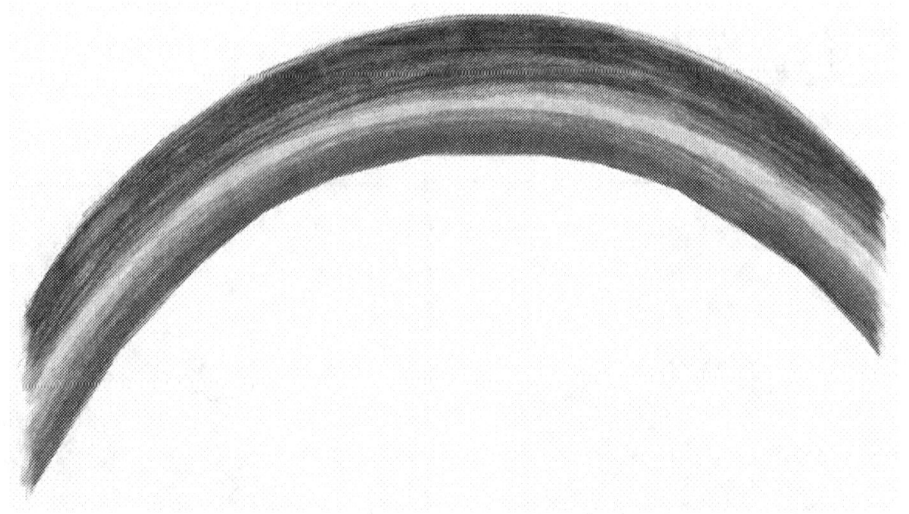

Neck & Shoulders

Chin Up
Chin Down

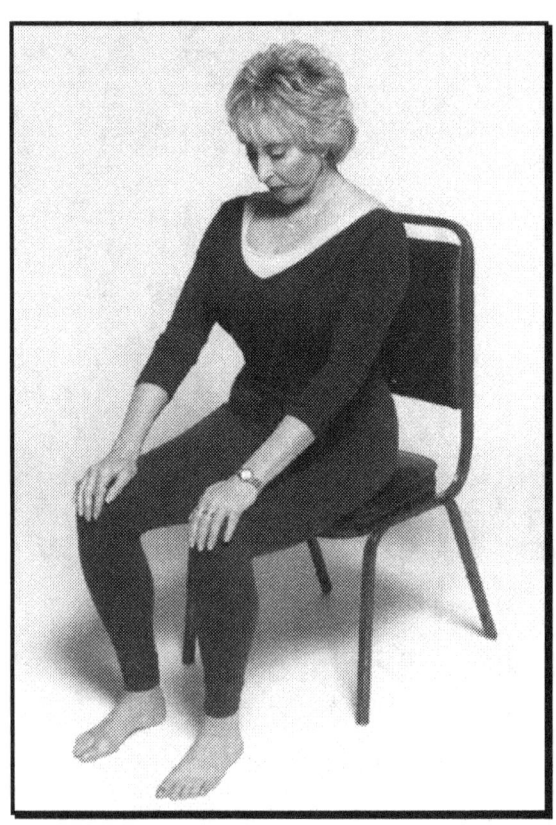
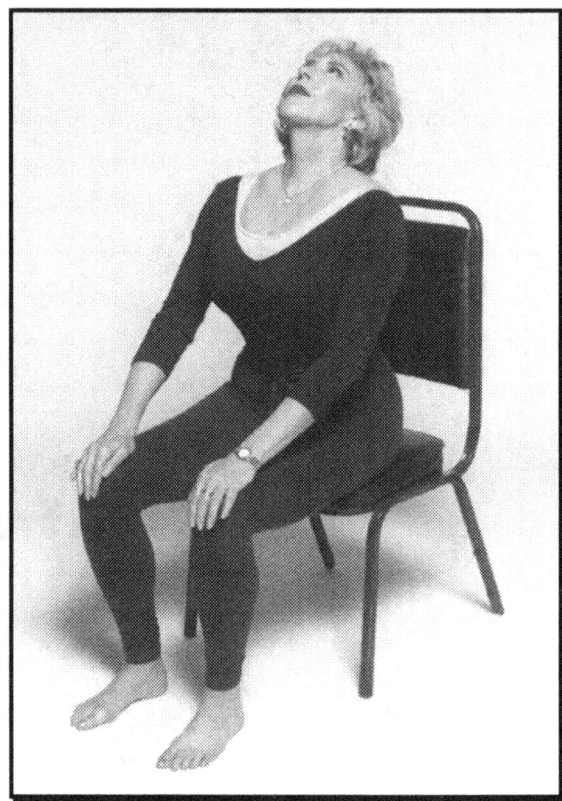

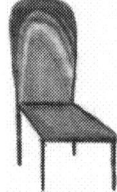 Sit tall in chair, shoulders down, chest up.

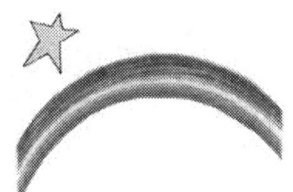

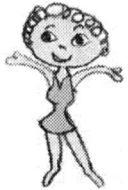 Raise chin gently tilting head back.

Lower chin slowly to chest.

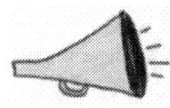 Comfortably repeat this movement - up and down.

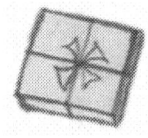 Easy does it!

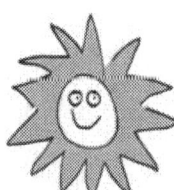

"I say 'yes!'
to good in my life."

Ear to Shoulder

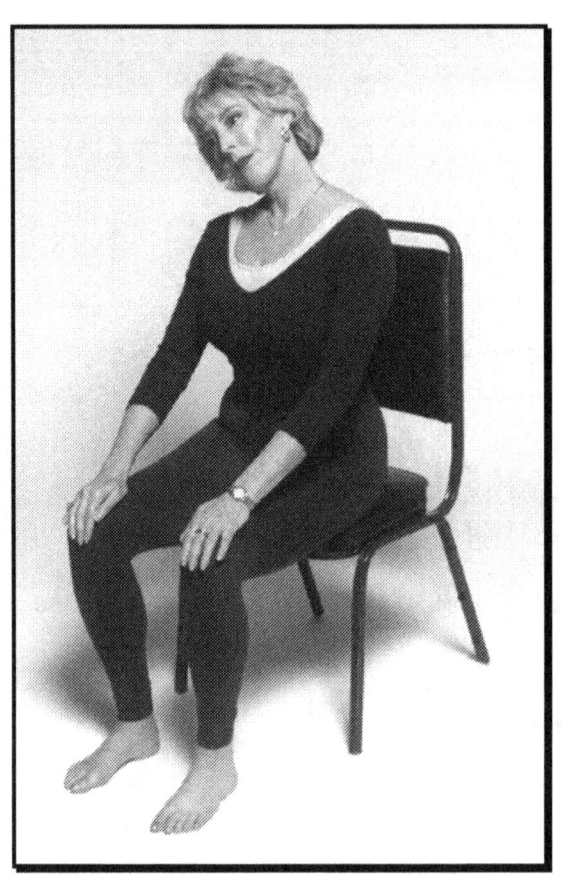 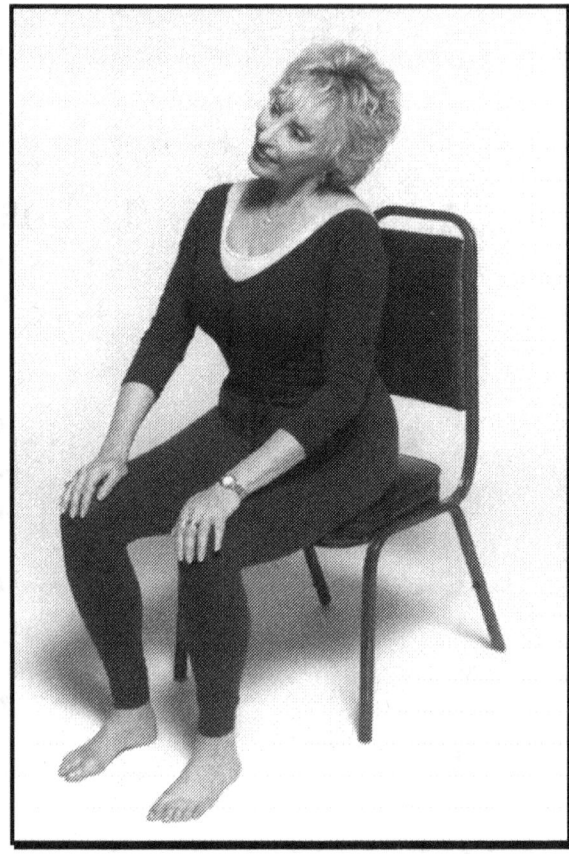

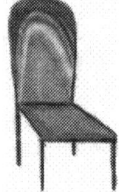 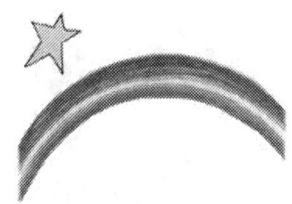 Sit tall in chair,
shoulders down,
chest up.
Look straight ahead.

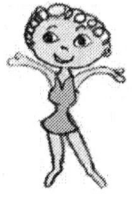 Gently tilt head
- ear to shoulder.

Return head to upright
position.

Now tilt head to other
shoulder.

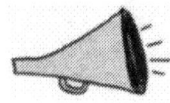 Repeat, relax and enjoy.

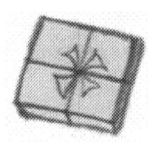 Keep it light!

"I listen to my body."

Face Left
Face Right

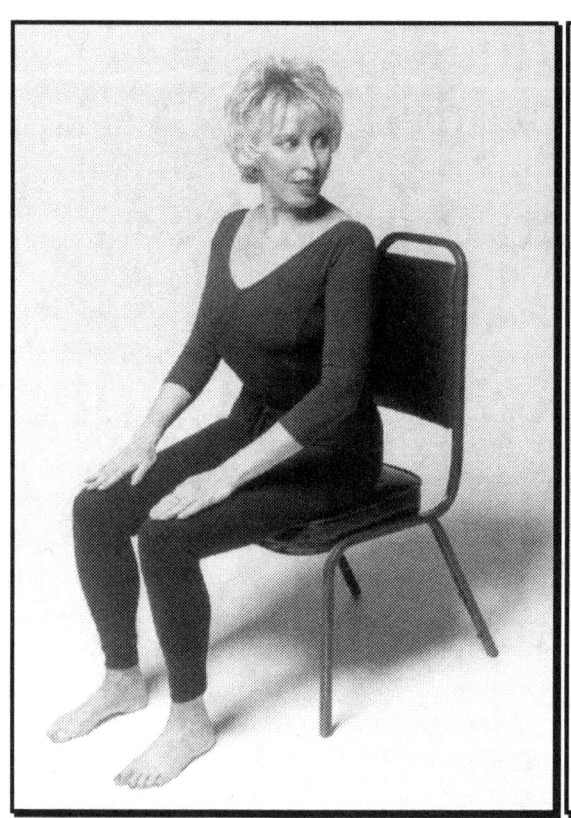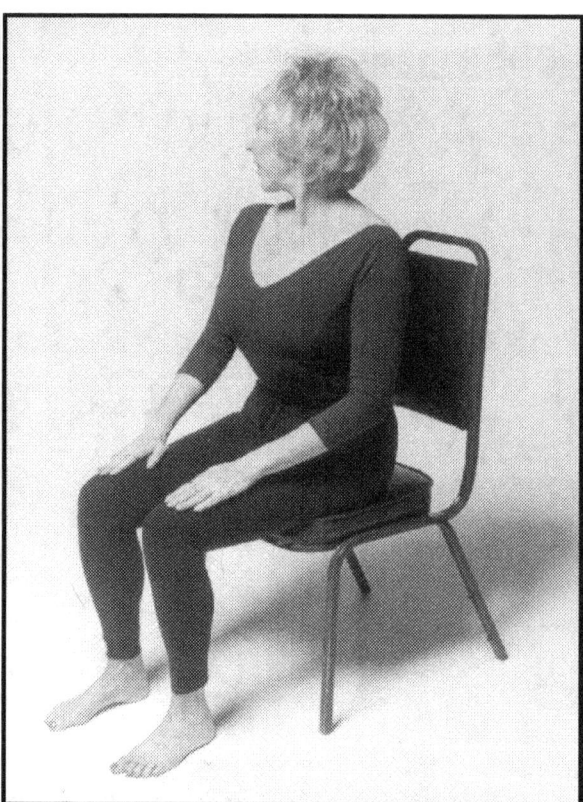

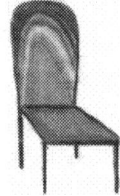 Sit tall in chair, shoulders down, chest up.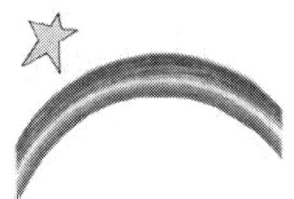

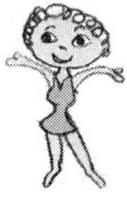 Gently look to the left.

Return to center.

Gently look to the right.

Return to center.

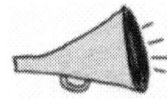 Repeat with confidence.

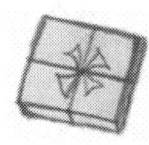 Looks great!

"I am not afraid to say 'no'."

Push Ahead

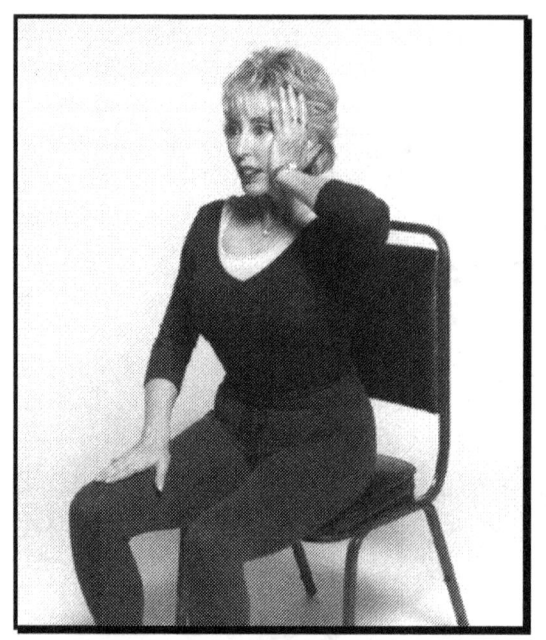
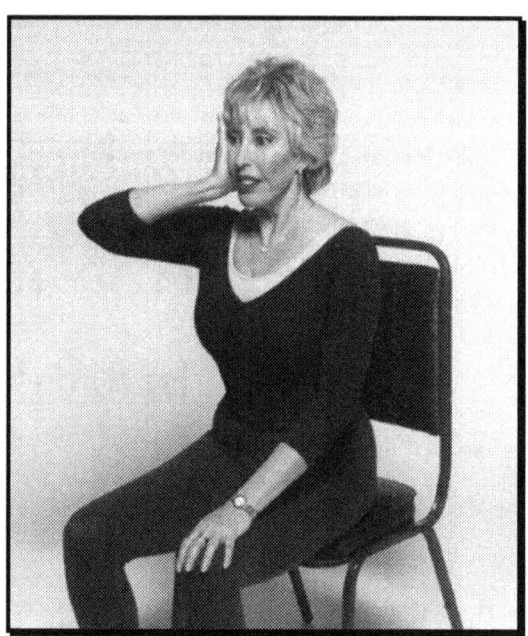
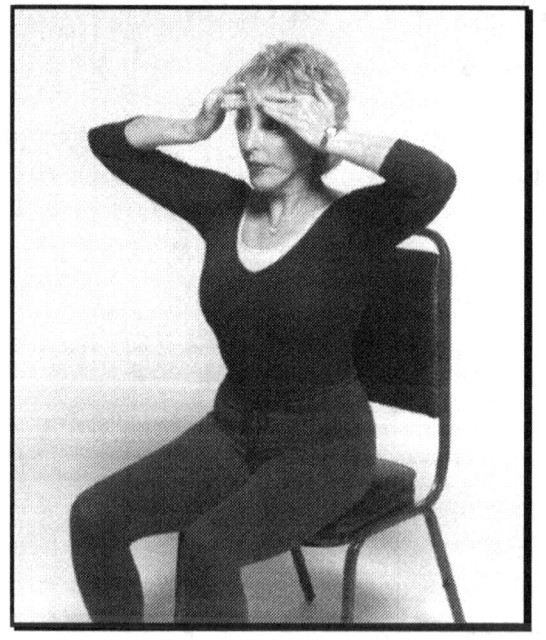
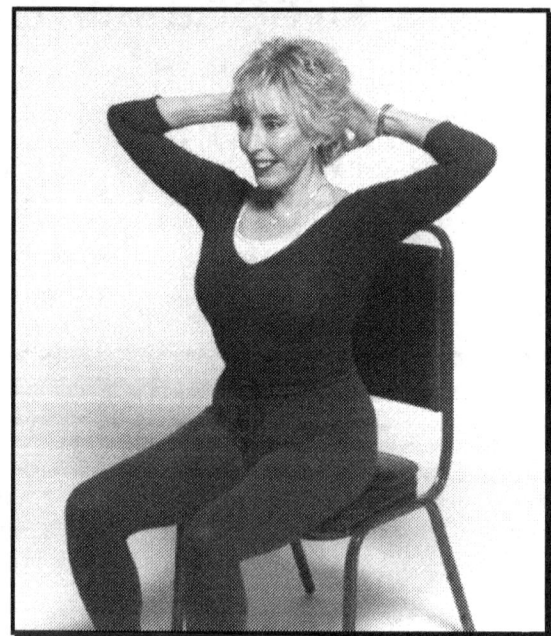

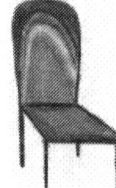 Sit tall in chair, shoulders down, chest up.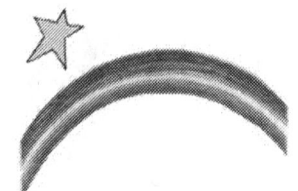

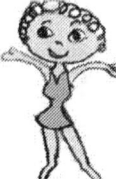 Push head into left palm.

Push head into right palm.

Press fingertips of both hands into forehead and hold.

Press fingertips of both hands into the back of head.

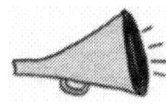 Keep head centered with resistance and gently repeat each movement several times.

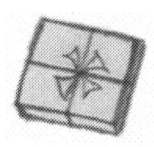 Smile!

"I press ahead in all areas of my life."

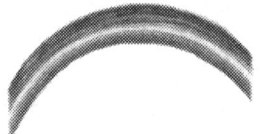

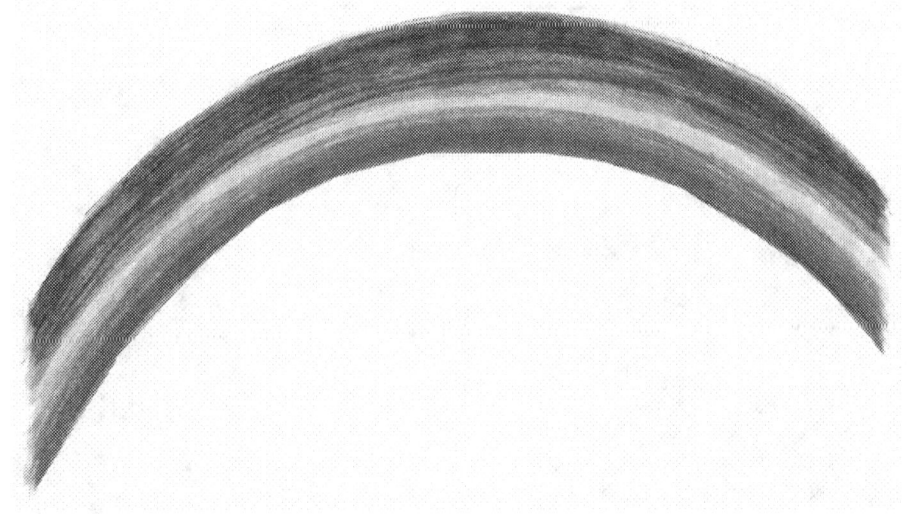

Shoulders &
Upper Back

Shoulder Lifts

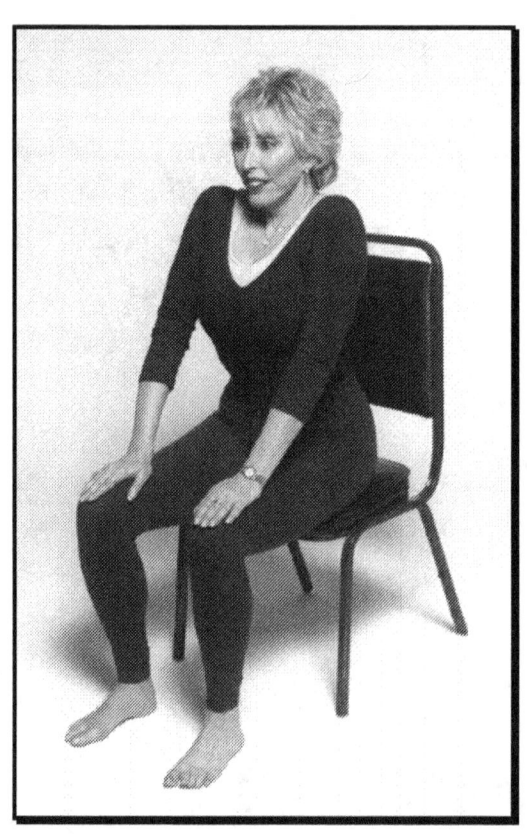 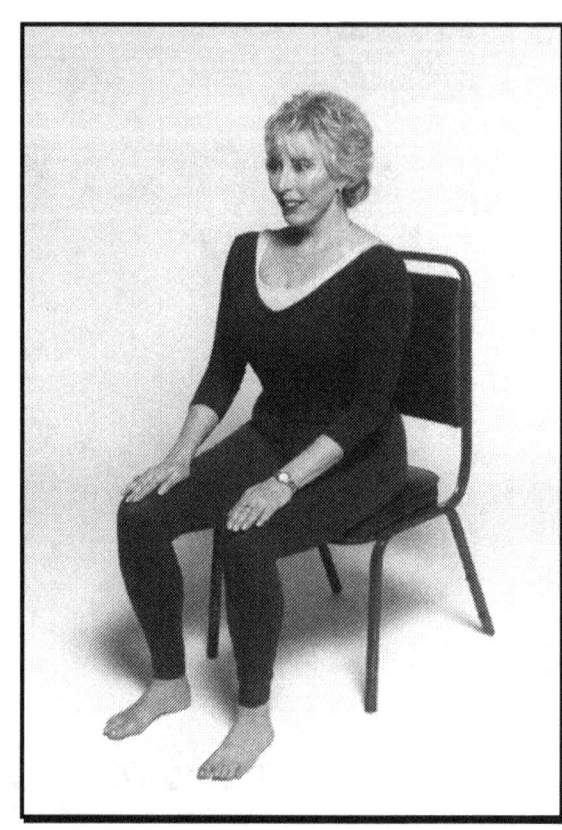

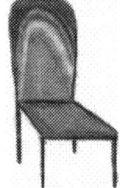 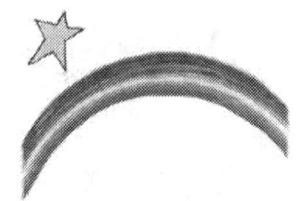 Sit tall in chair,
shoulders down,
chest up.
Rest arms on thighs.

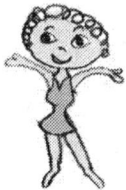 Lift shoulders up to ears
- inhale.

Slowly drop shoulders,
relax - exhale.

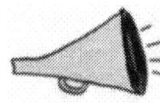 Repeat joyously.

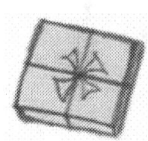 Having fun is good!

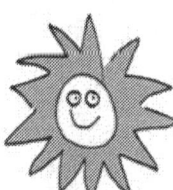

"I shrug off the blues."

Shoulder &
Arm Stretch

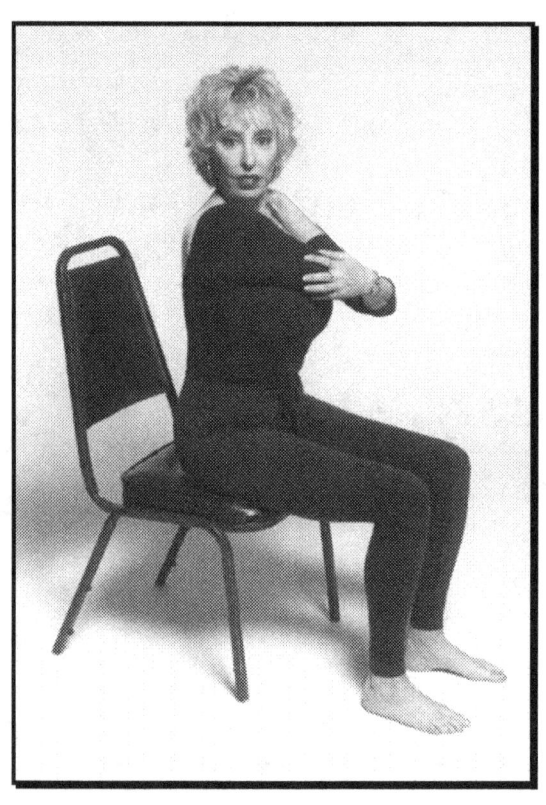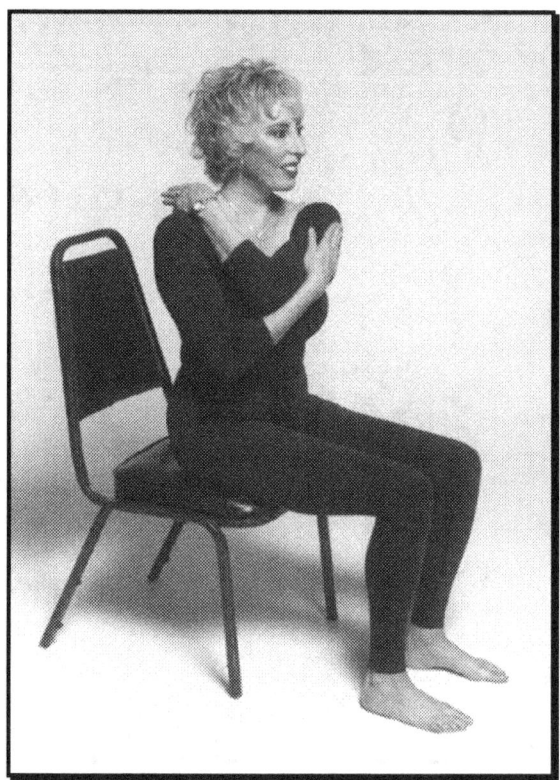

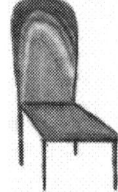 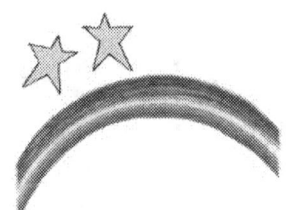 Sit tall in chair, shoulders down, chest up.

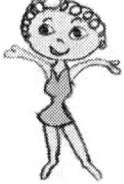 With one arm, reach around the other and place the hand near the top part of the shoulder.

With the other arm, reach up and gently pull the elbow across the chest.

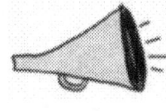 Repeat on other side. That feels good!

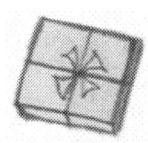 Give yourself a hug!

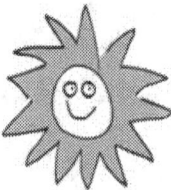

"I hold myself dear."

Shoulder Drop

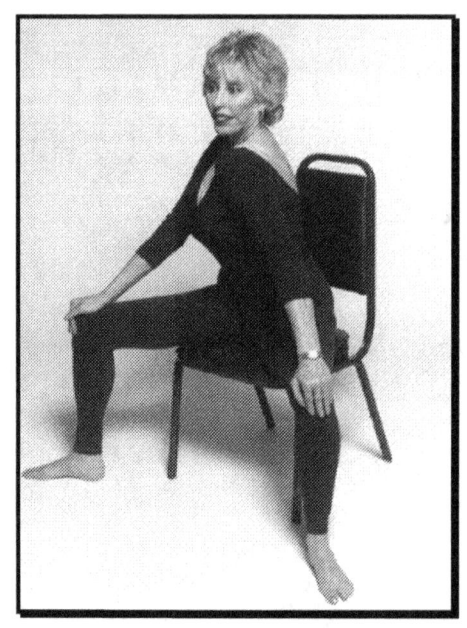
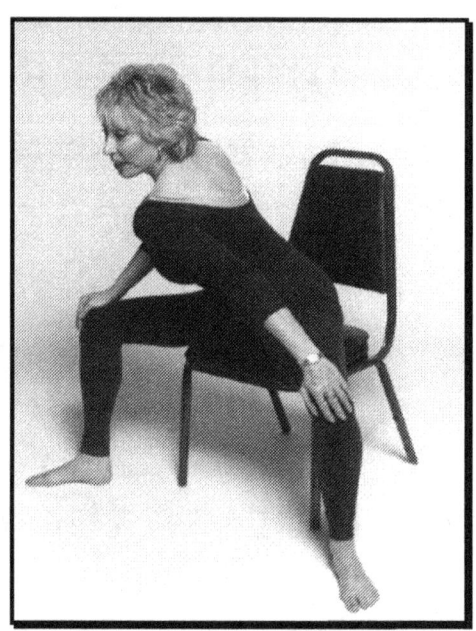
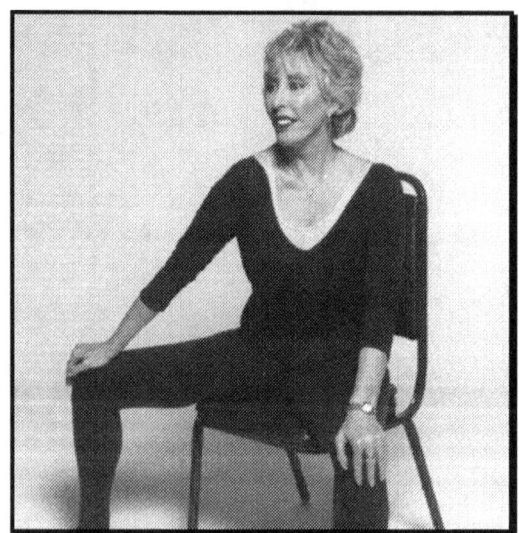
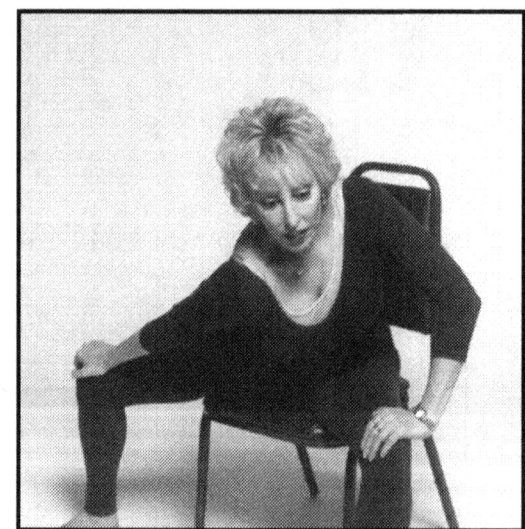

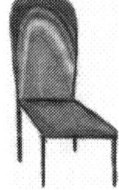  Sit tall at the edge of chair, shoulders down, chest up. Separate legs and feet as far as comfortable.

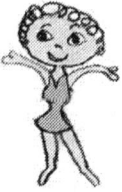 Place hands on thighs and slowly drop one shoulder forward to opposite knee.

Gently stretch.

Change to the other side.

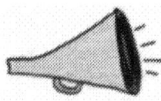 Keep head in a neutral position and repeat the stretch.

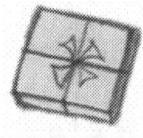 Feeling great!

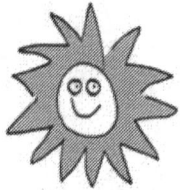

"I gracefully shoulder all life's challenges."

Chain Breaker

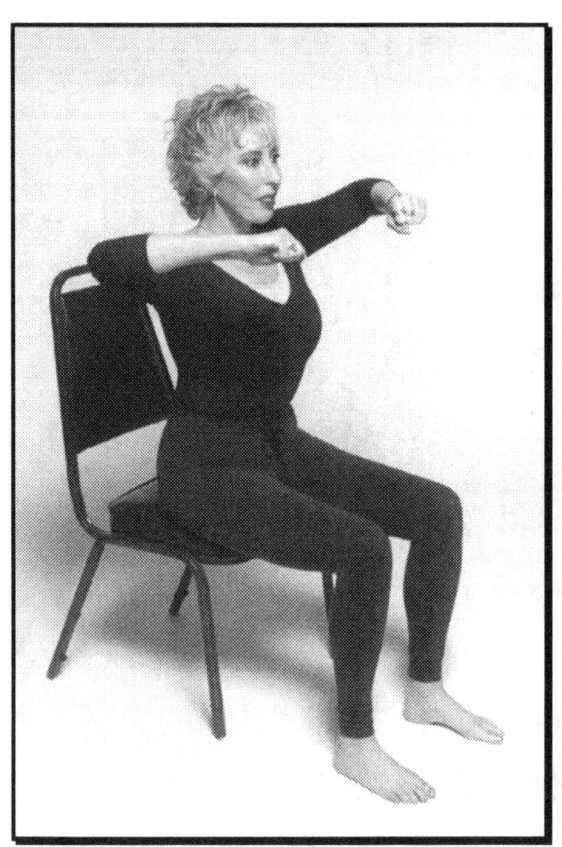 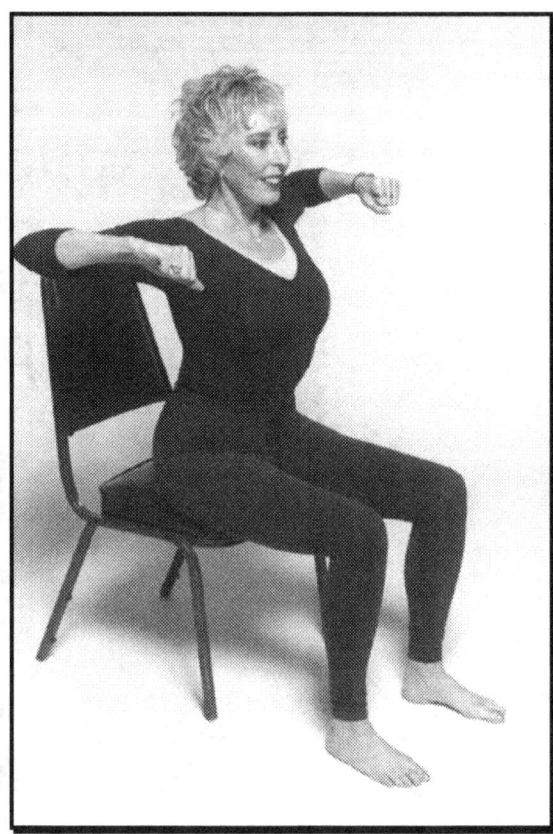

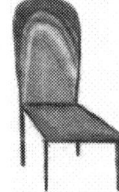 Sit tall in chair, shoulders down, chest up.

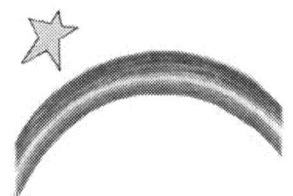

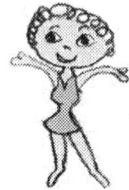 Place fists together - elbows raised.

Gently press both arms back.

"Break the chain."

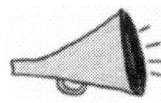 Repeat with glee.

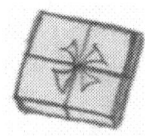 Looking good!

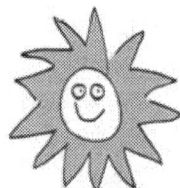

"I open myself to the love that surrounds me."

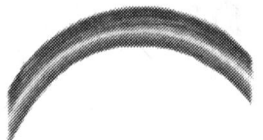

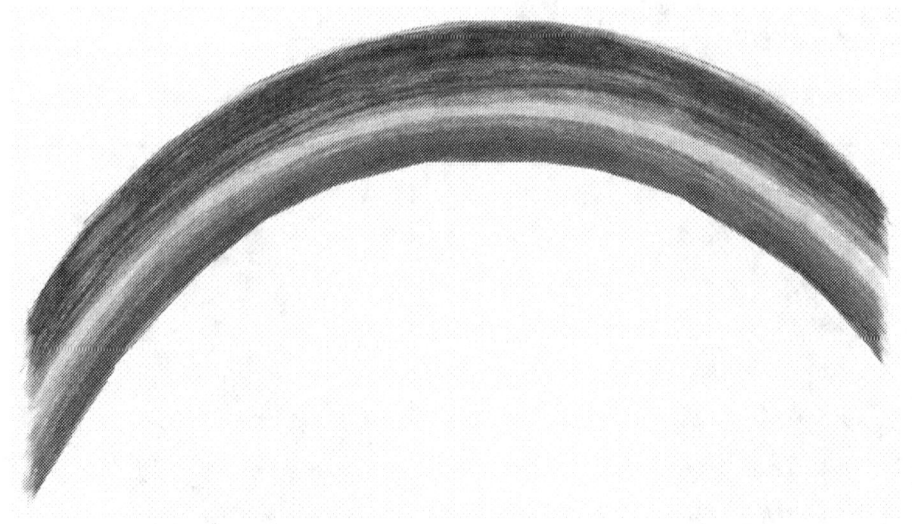

Arms &
Upper Back

Overhead Elbow Pull

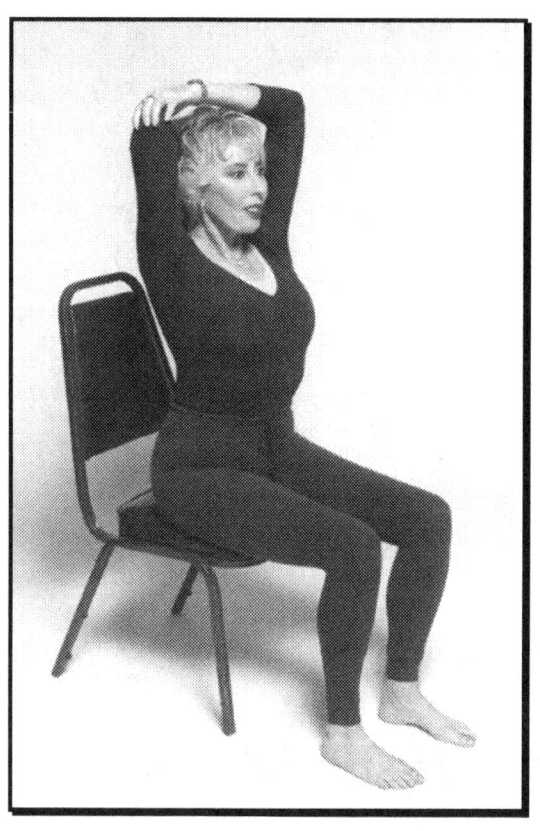 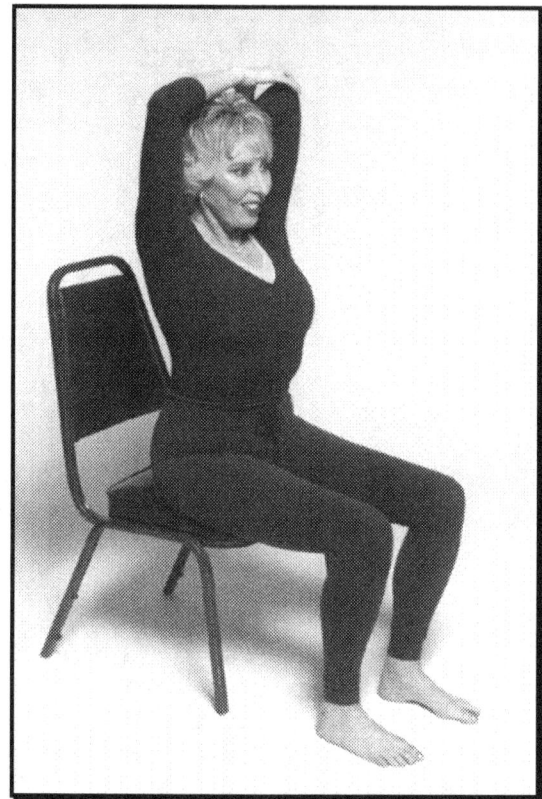

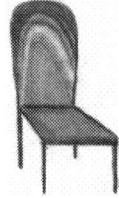 Sit tall in chair, shoulders down, chest up.

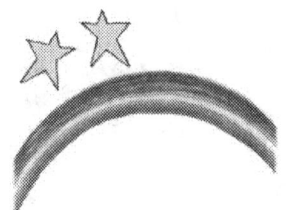

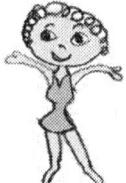 Lift both arms above head.

Hold bent elbow of one arm.

Keeping the head even, stretch the back of the arm by gently pressing the elbow with the opposite hand.

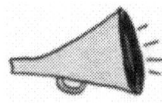 Repeat with the other arm.

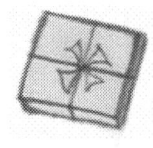 Nice!

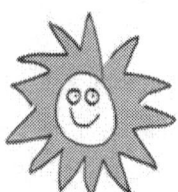

"I love my body."

Peck Up

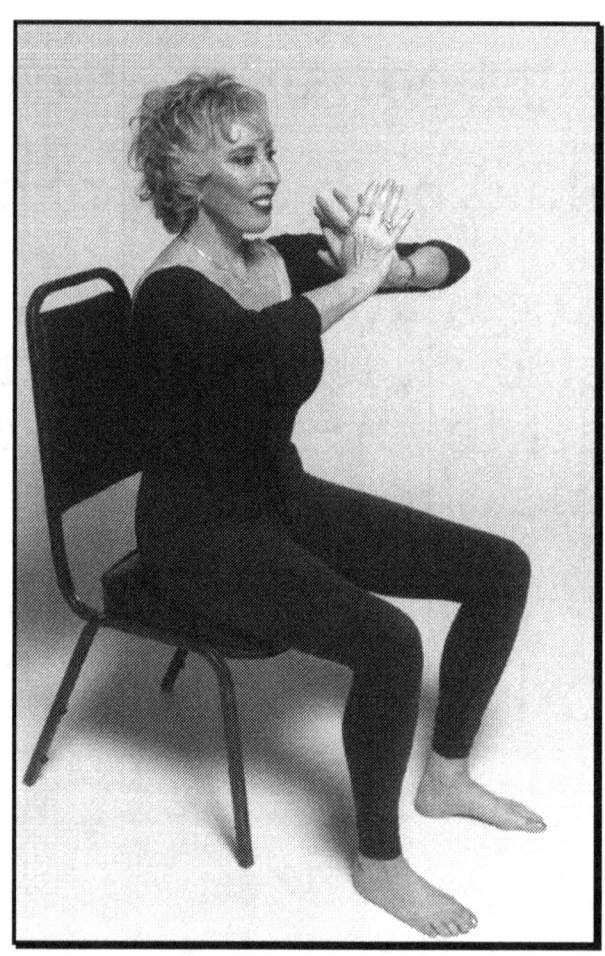

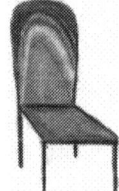 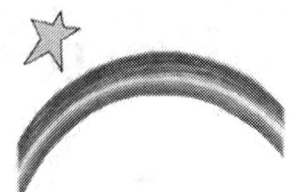 Sit tall in chair, shoulders down, chest up.

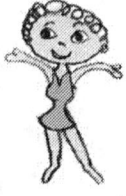 Inhale.

Press hands together in front of chest.

Exhale.

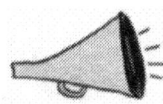 Repeat thankfully.

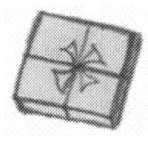 Bravo!

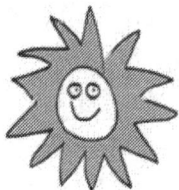

"I join in peace, love and laughter."

Reach Out

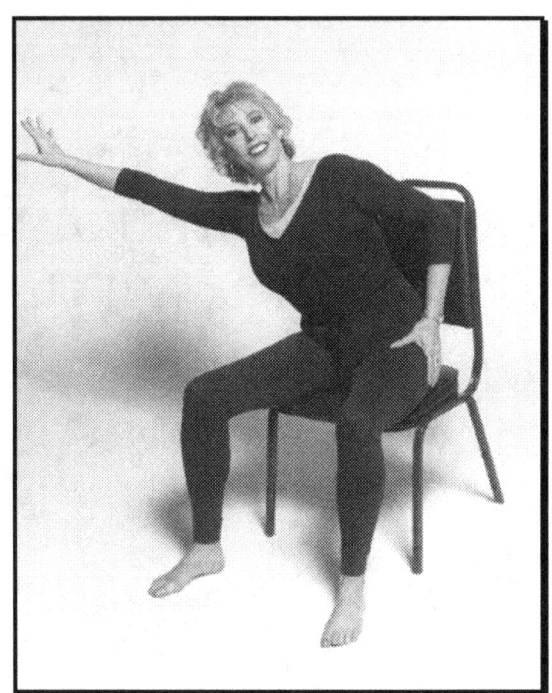 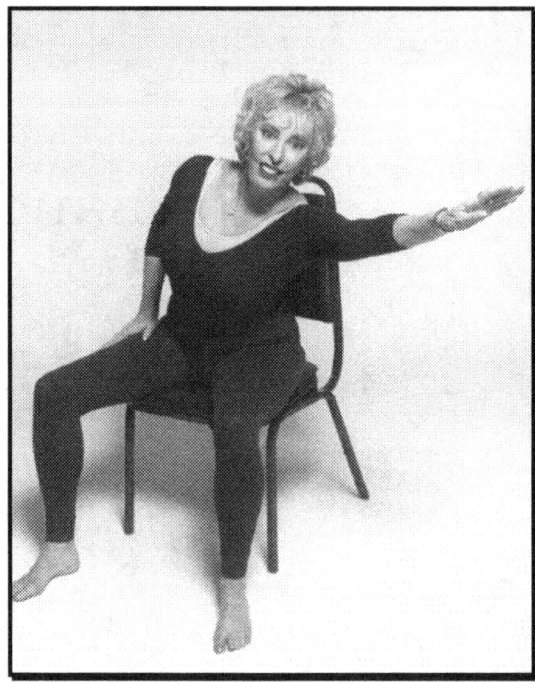

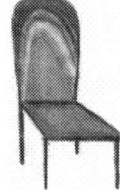 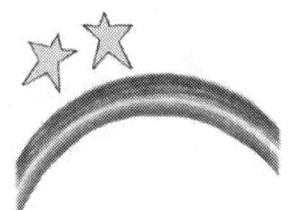 Sit tall in chair, shoulders down, chest up, legs shoulder-width apart, stomach in.

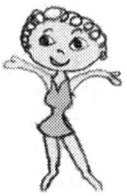 Gently reach arm out to the side, palm down, in a flowing motion.

Stretch body.

Alternate side to side in a flowing motion.

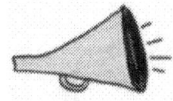 Repeat lovingly.

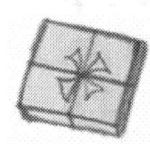 Easy does it!

"I reach out in loving ways to all I meet."

Reach High

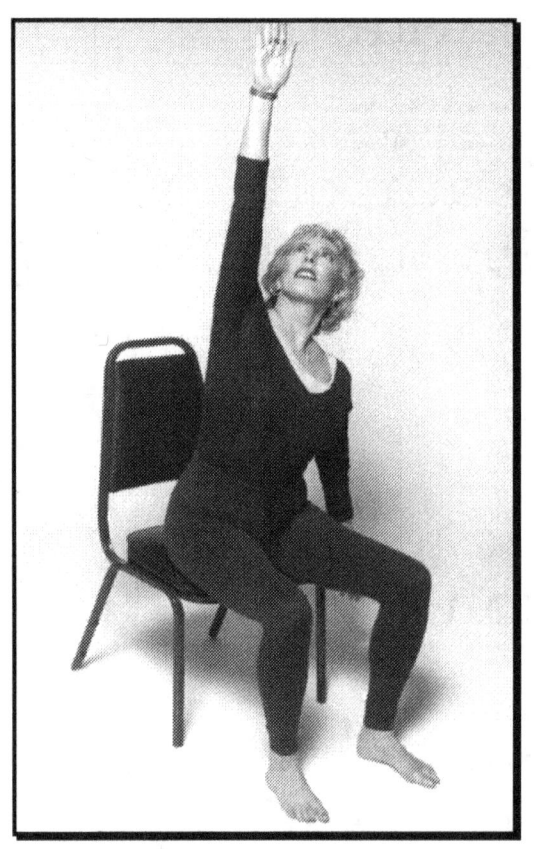 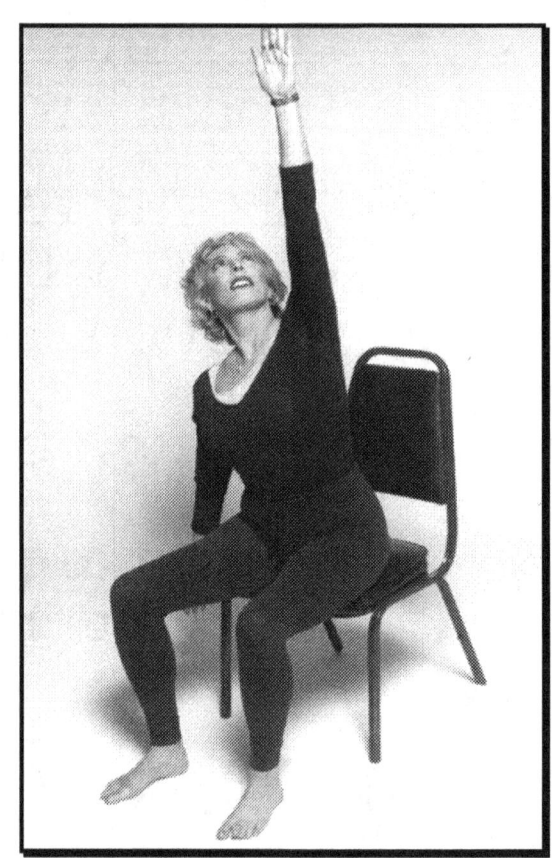

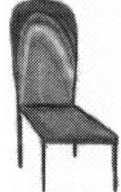 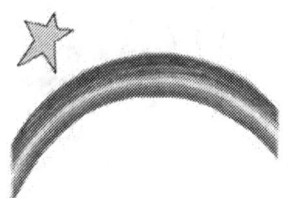 Sit tall in chair, shoulders down, chest up. Relax one arm to the side.

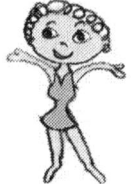 Gently stretch as you reach upward with the opposite arm.

Look at fingertips as you extend the arm upward.

Repeat on other side.

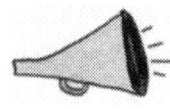 Alternate the stretch on each side.

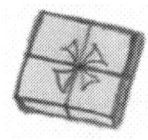 Exercise is fun!

"I reach for my highest good."

Reach Higher

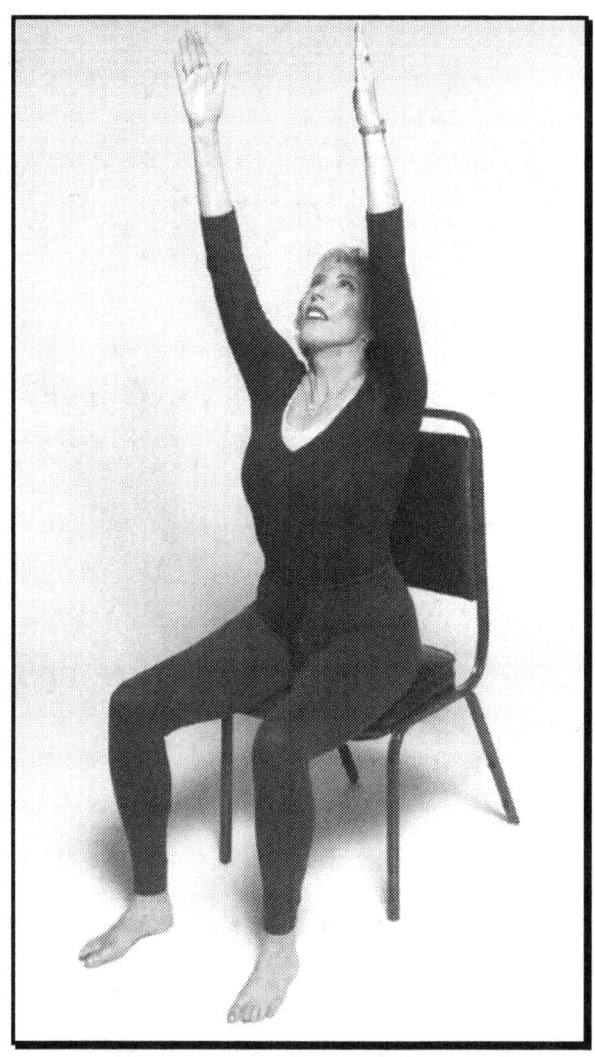

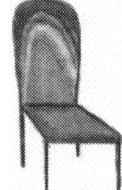 Sit tall in chair, shoulders down, chest up, with legs shoulder-width apart, stomach in.

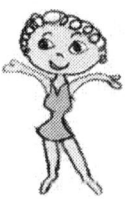 Gently lift both arms overhead - inhale.

Slowly lower arms – exhale.

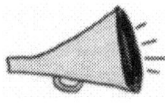 Repeat comfortably.

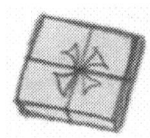 Reach for the stars!

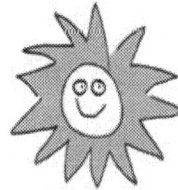

"Each and every day
I reach for my rainbow."

Rope Climb

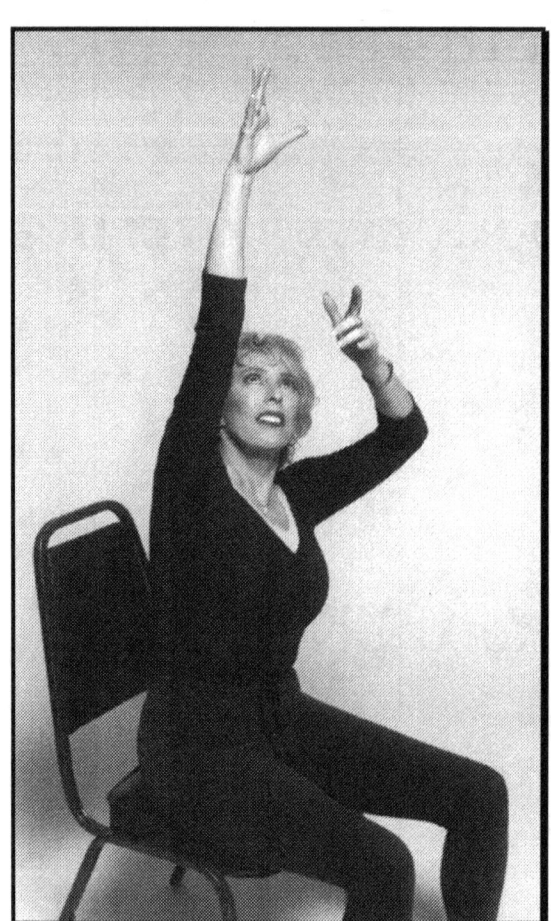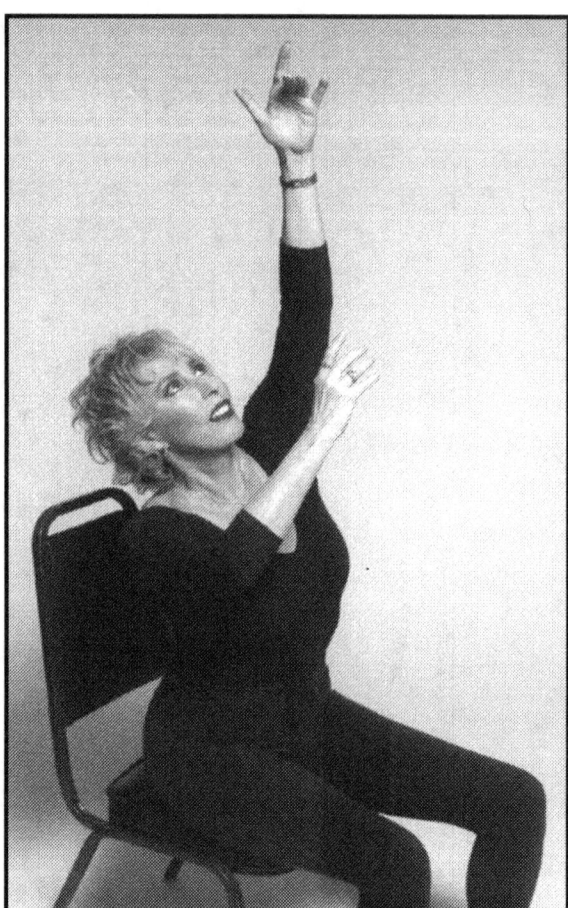

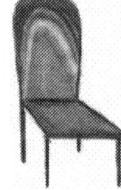
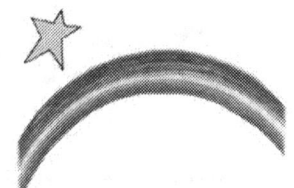

Sit tall in chair, shoulders down, chest up.

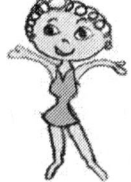

Raise one arm up as if scaling a rope.

Pull yourself up the imaginary rope one hand after the other.

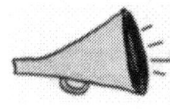

Continue climbing the rope until you reach the top.

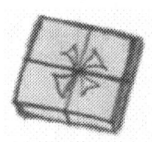

I'm proud of you!

"I enjoy the journey and set my sights high."

Beach Ball

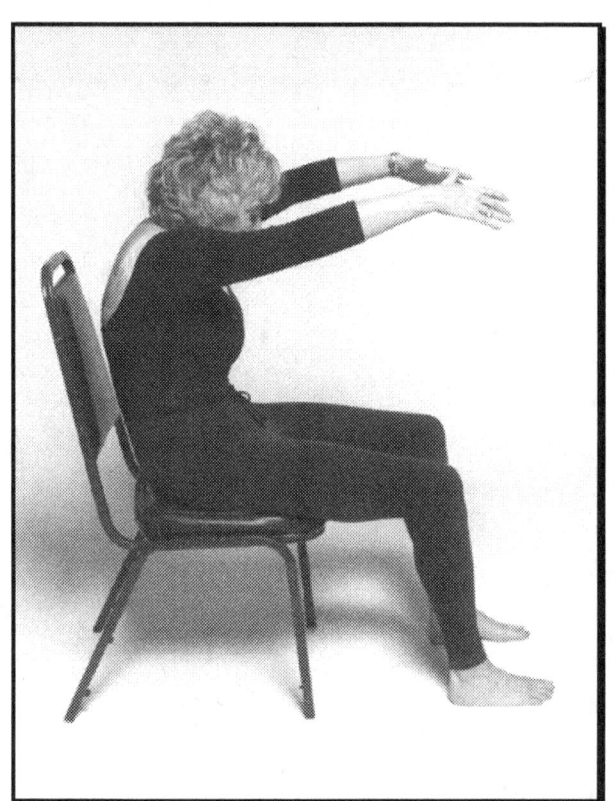 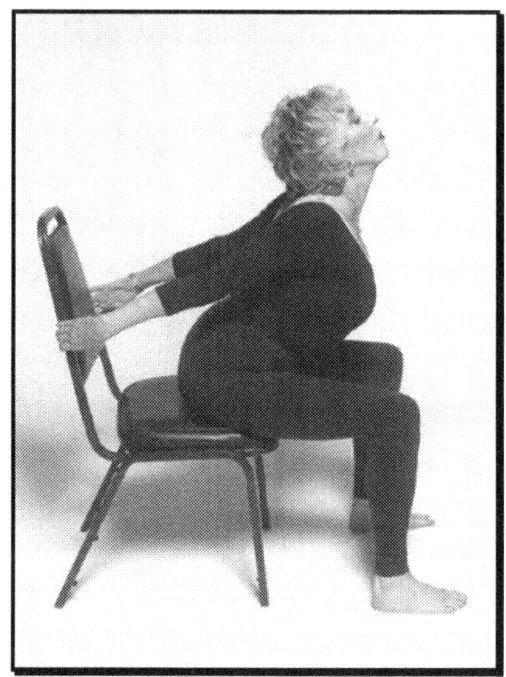

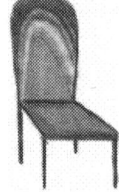 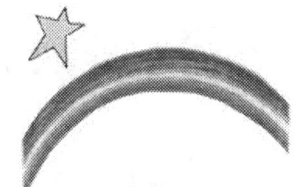 Sit tall in chair, shoulders down, chest up.

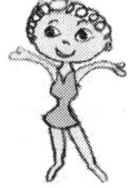 Round back as you extend both arms outward as if hugging a large beach ball – exhale.

Then, reach hands to back of chair gently arching the back –inhale.

Press chest forward, shoulders back.

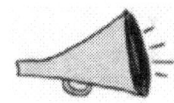 Comfortably repeat.

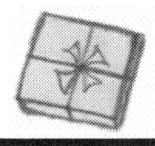 Have a ball!

"I embrace the world and reach out with love."

Swaying Side Stretch (One Arm)

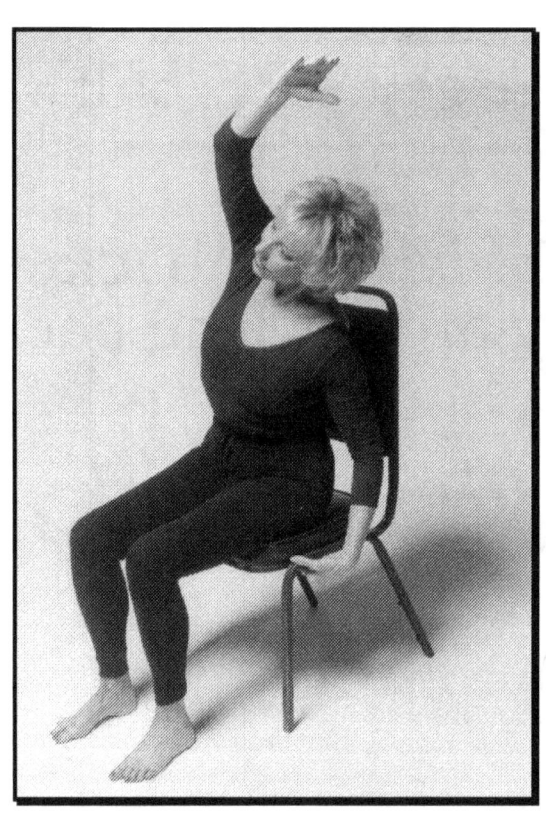 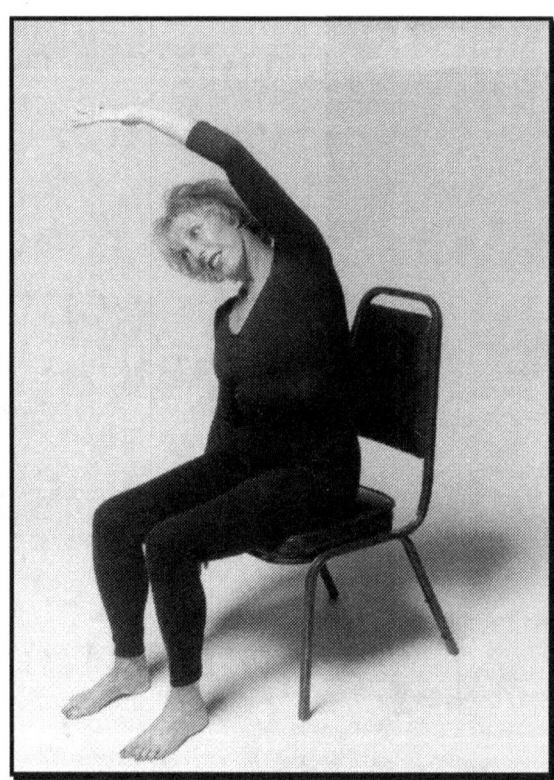

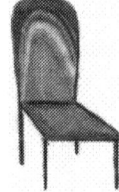 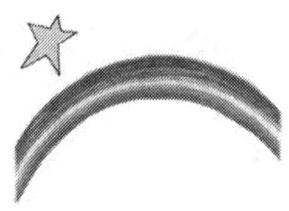 Sit tall in chair,
shoulders down,
chest up, with feet
shoulder-width apart.

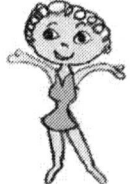 Lift one arm above head.

Gently stretch to the side.

Switch arms.

Sway to the other side and
stretch.

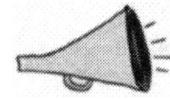 Repeat.

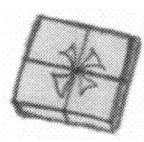 Good show!

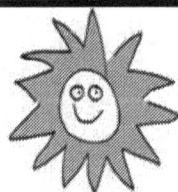

*"I sway like a tree
and sing with each season."*

Swaying Side Stretch

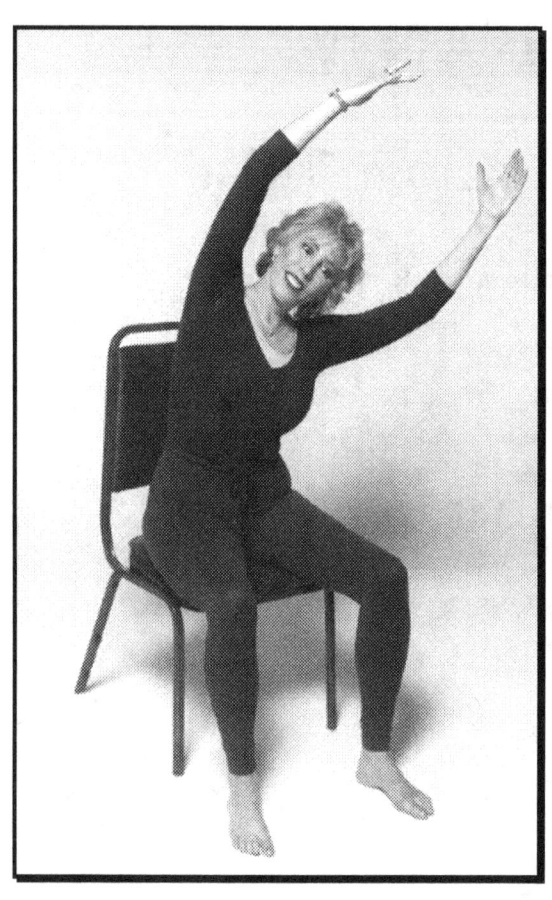 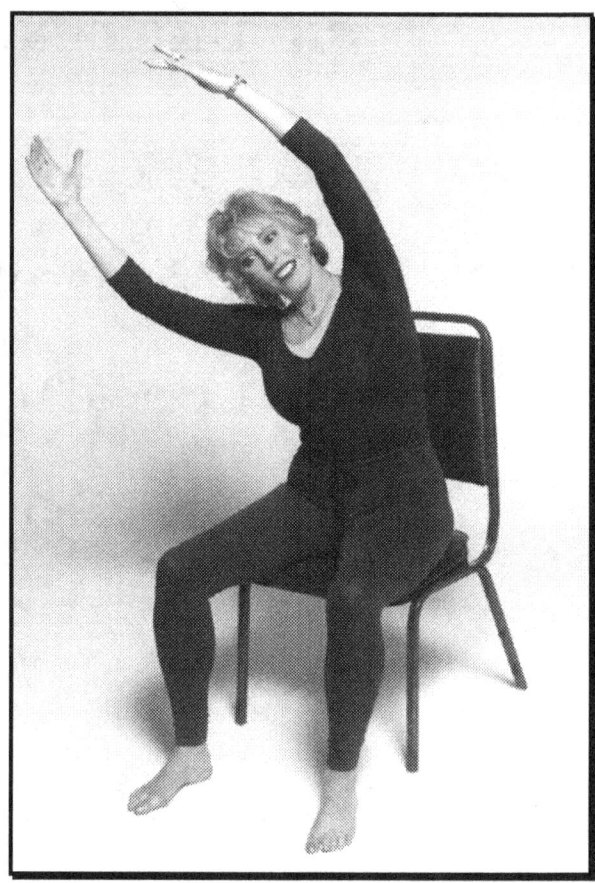

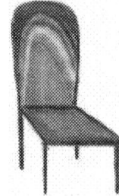 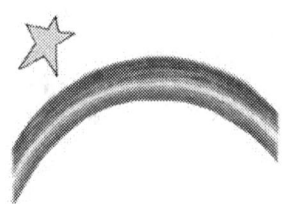 Sit tall in chair, shoulders down, chest up, with feet shoulder-width apart.

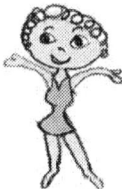 Lift both arms above head.

Stretch to the side.

Sway to the other side and stretch.

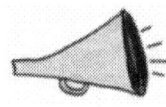 Repeat gracefully.

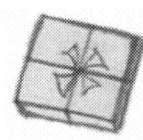 You're beautiful!

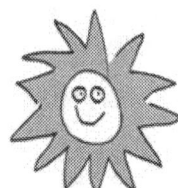

"I am flexible and free."

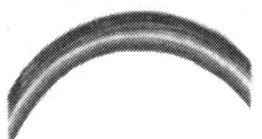

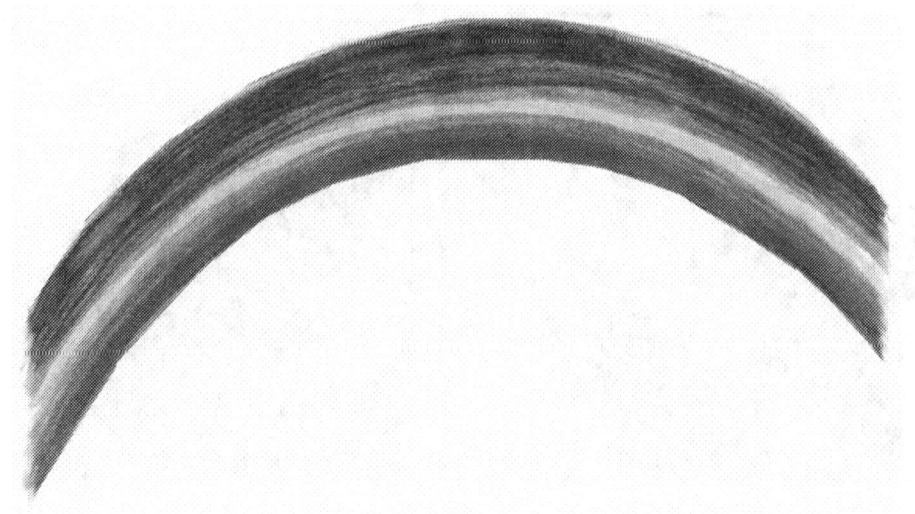

Arms, Hands & Wrists

Wrist Stretch

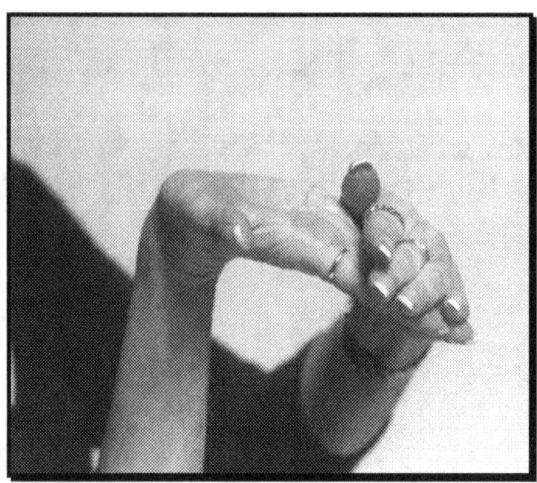 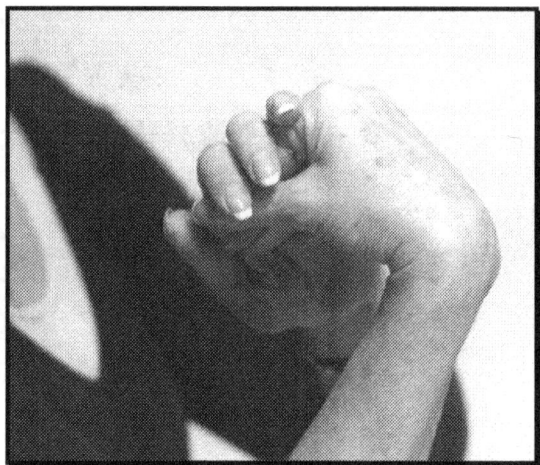

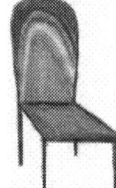 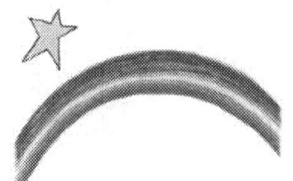 Sit tall in chair, shoulders down, chest up.
Bend arms upward to place hands in front of chest.

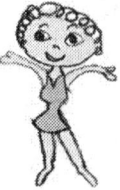 First, place one hand palm up and gently press fingers back with other hand.

Next, gently bend hand toward you and press down on the tops of fingers.

Change hands and stretch other wrist back and forth as above.

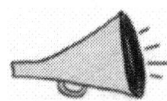 Repeat comfortably

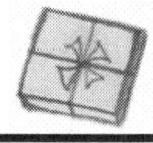 Give yourself a hand!

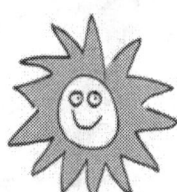

"I appreciate and respect myself."

Finger Stretch

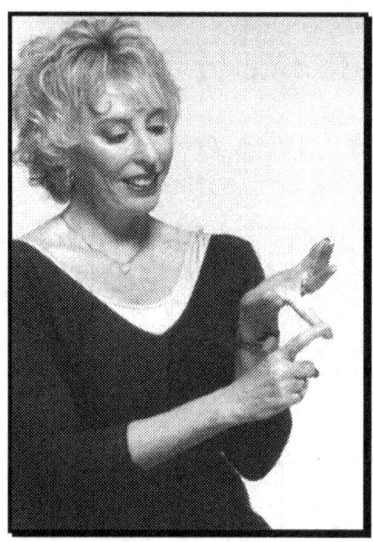

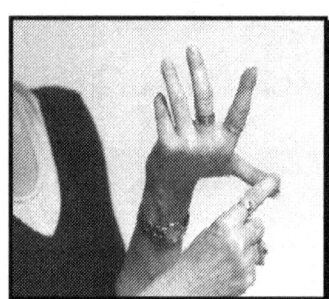
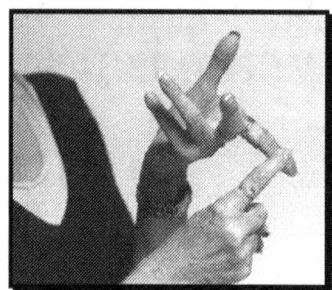
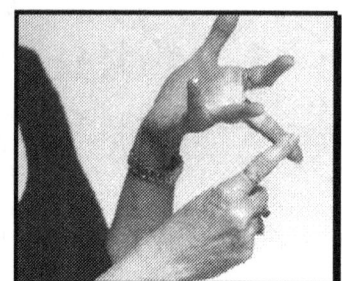

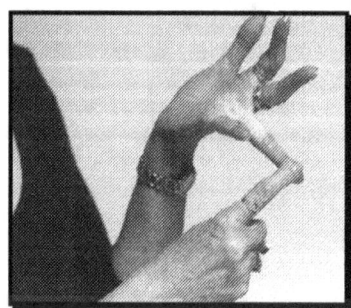
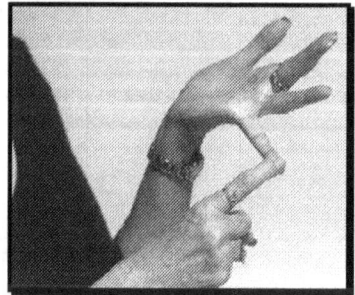

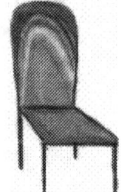 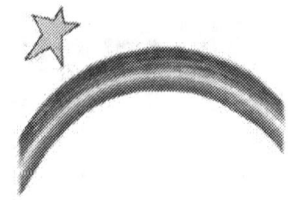 Sit tall in chair, shoulders down, chest up.
Keep elbows close to body.

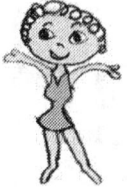 With one hand, palm up, grasp the thumb and gently stretch it downward.

Repeat this motion for each finger.

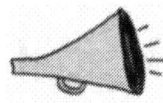 Repeat with other hand.

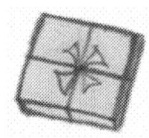 This little piggy...

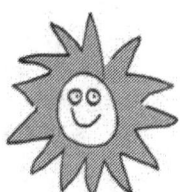

"All life's details work out with ease."

Wrist Flip Flops

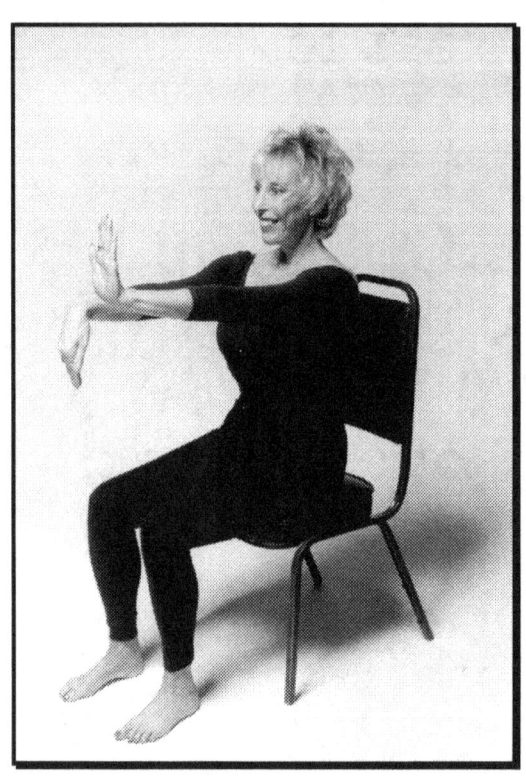 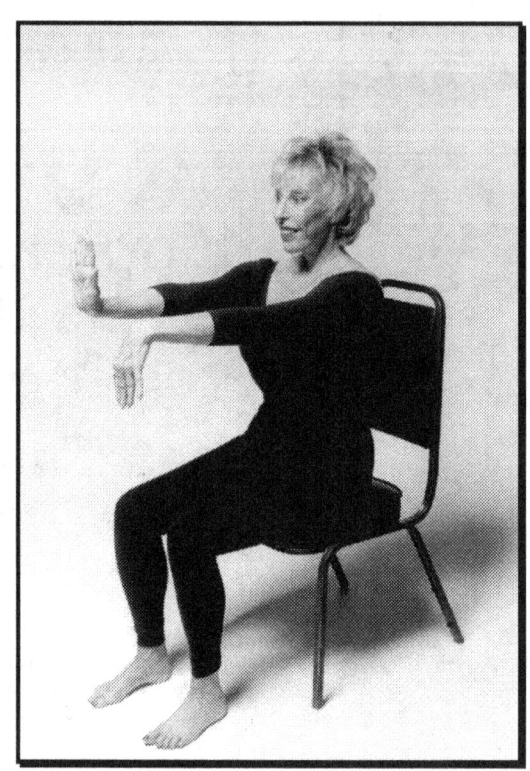

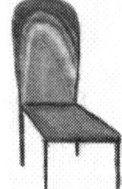 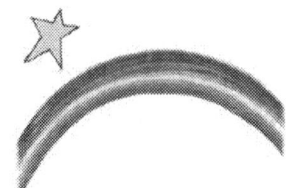 Sit tall in chair, shoulders down, chest up. Extend arms parallel to floor and relax wrists.

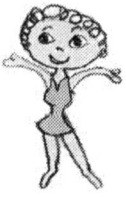 Keep both arms out parallel to floor.

Raise one hand, wrist bent back, fingers to ceiling.

Alternate position with one hand, raising it as you drop the other.

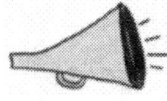 Keep your arms straight.

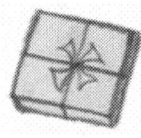 Flip Flop. You're on top!

"Goodbye to the blues -
hello to happiness."

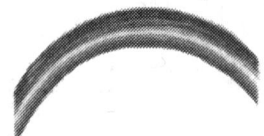

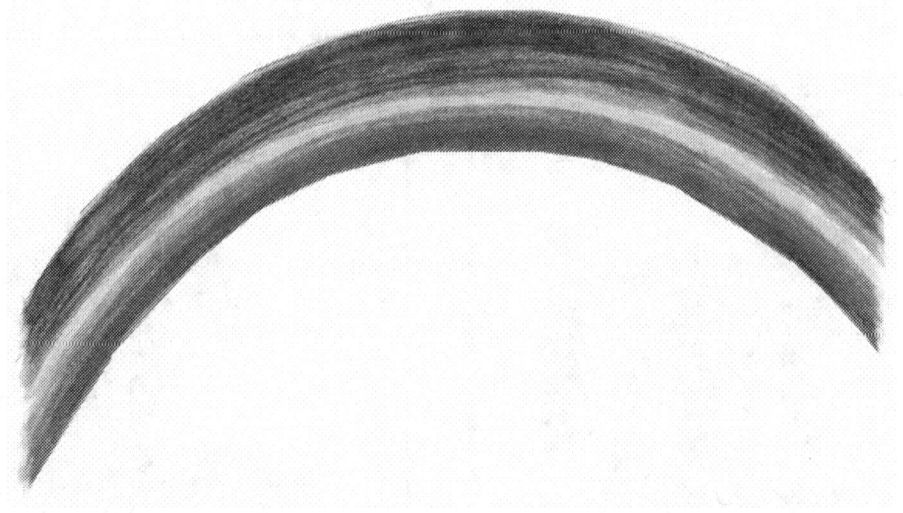

Upper & Lower Back

Waist Bend

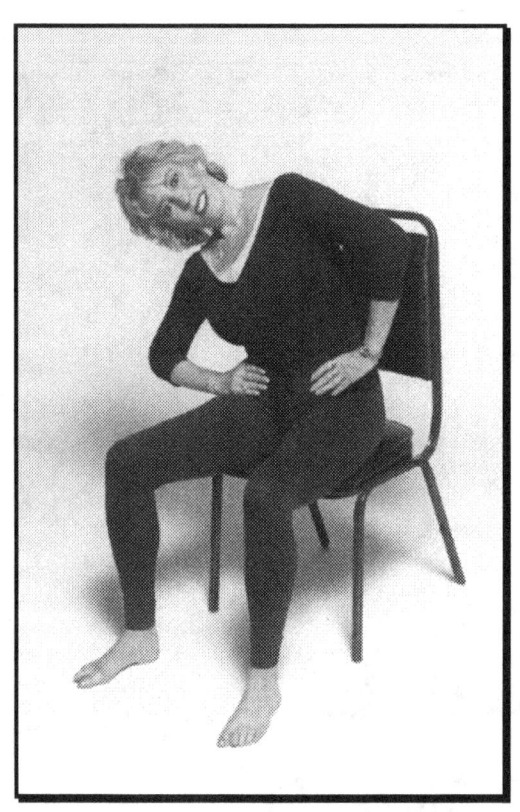 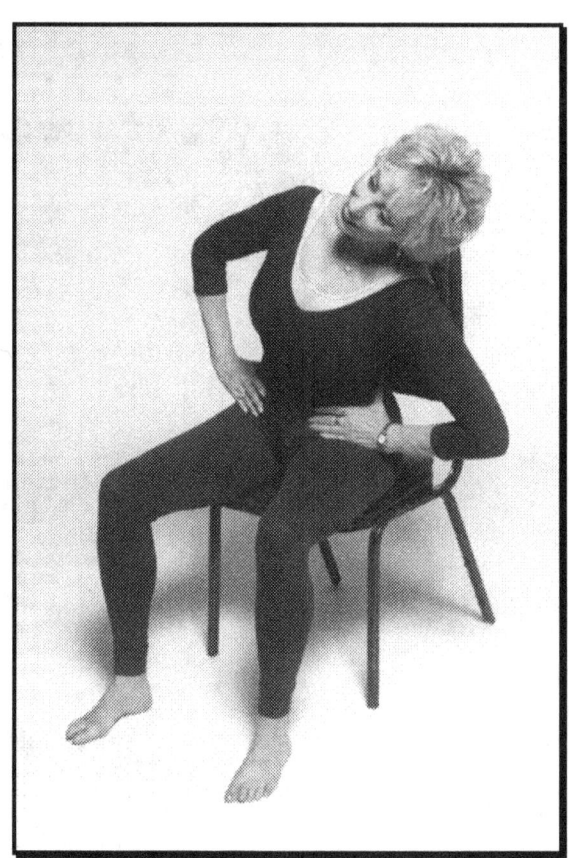

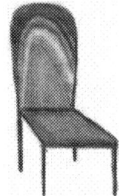 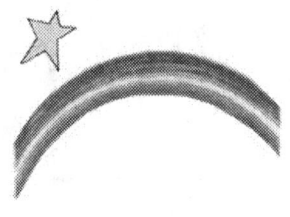 Sit tall in chair, shoulders down, chest up, with legs shoulder-width apart.

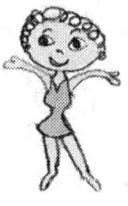 Place both hands on hips and gently lean to one side.

Sway to the other side.

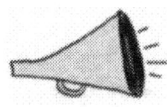 Repeat gracefully.

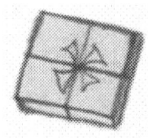 Excellent!

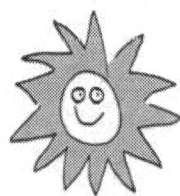

"I lean to love."

Bend & Reach

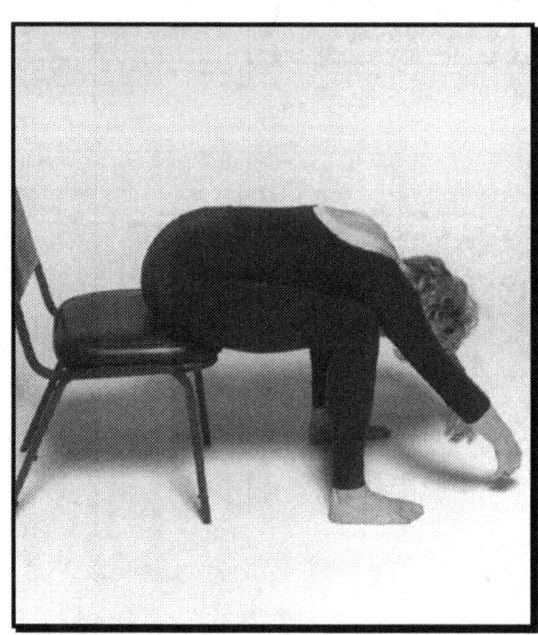 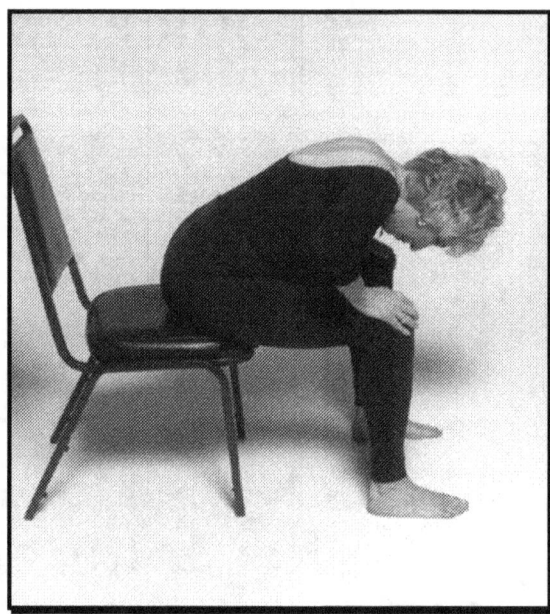

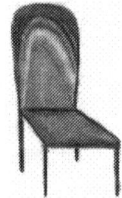  Sit tall in chair,
shoulders down,
chest up,
with hands on knees.

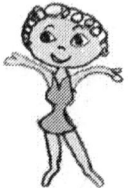 Gently bend forward to the floor.

Extend arms and head forward as far as is comfortable – exhale.

Place hands on knees for support as needed - inhale and lift body to upright position.

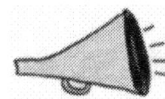 Repeat cheerfully.

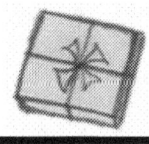 Doing good!

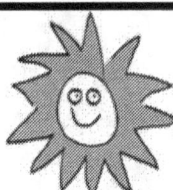

"I celebrate life's ups and downs."

Standing Side Bend

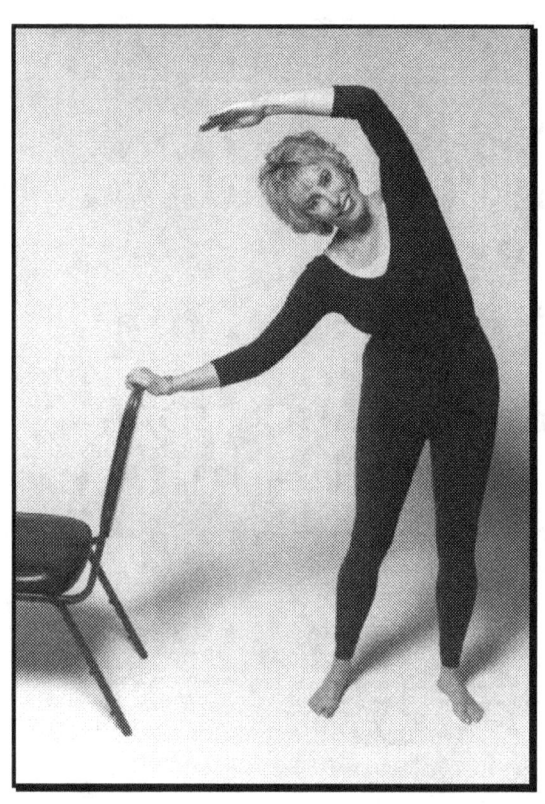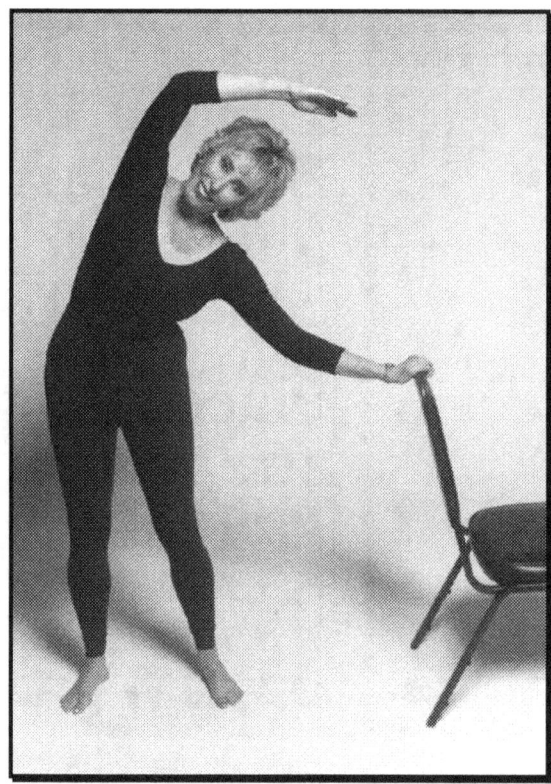

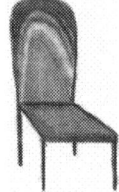 Stand tall beside chair, shoulders down, chest up. Place one hand on chair back for support.

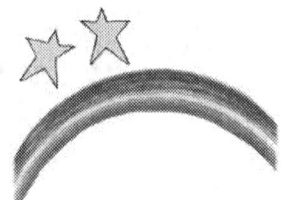

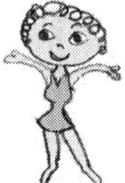 Reach opposite arm over head and gently bend toward the chair.

Turn and repeat this motion on the other side.

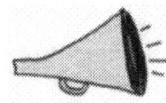 Repeat joyously.

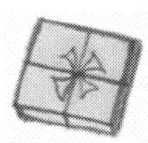 Doing good!

"I am flexible in my outlook on life."

Flat Back

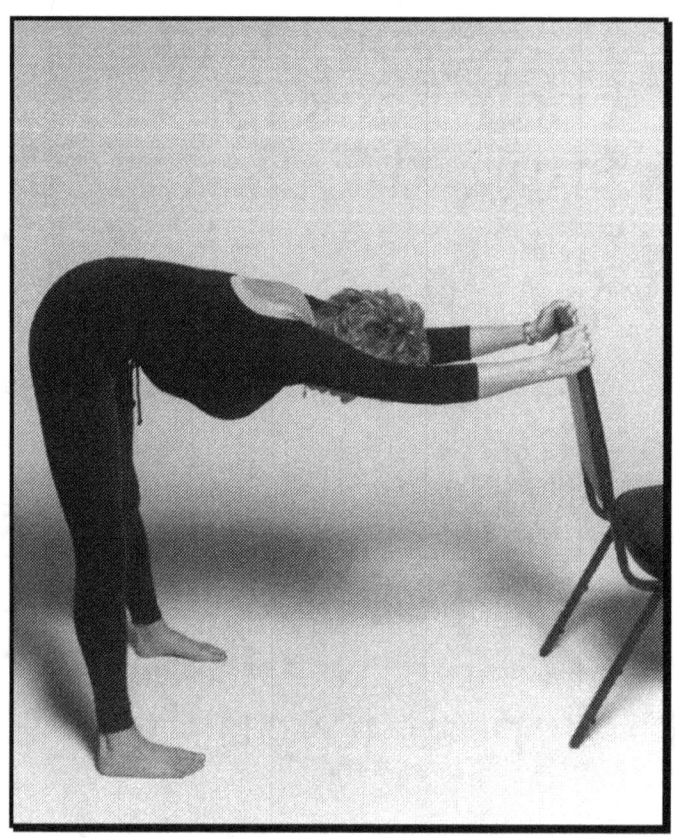

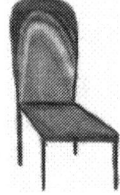

Stand behind chair at arms length. Place both hands on chair back, feet straight-ahead, hip-width apart.

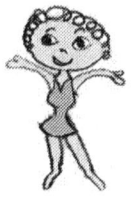

Gently lower upper torso, relax down.

Release all tension.

Bend knees and slowly roll up.

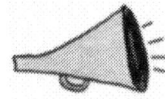

Repeat comfortably.

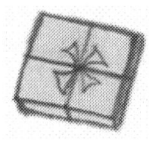

Nice Job!

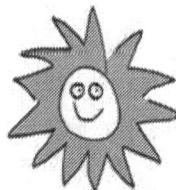

"I stretch to new horizons."

Lean Back

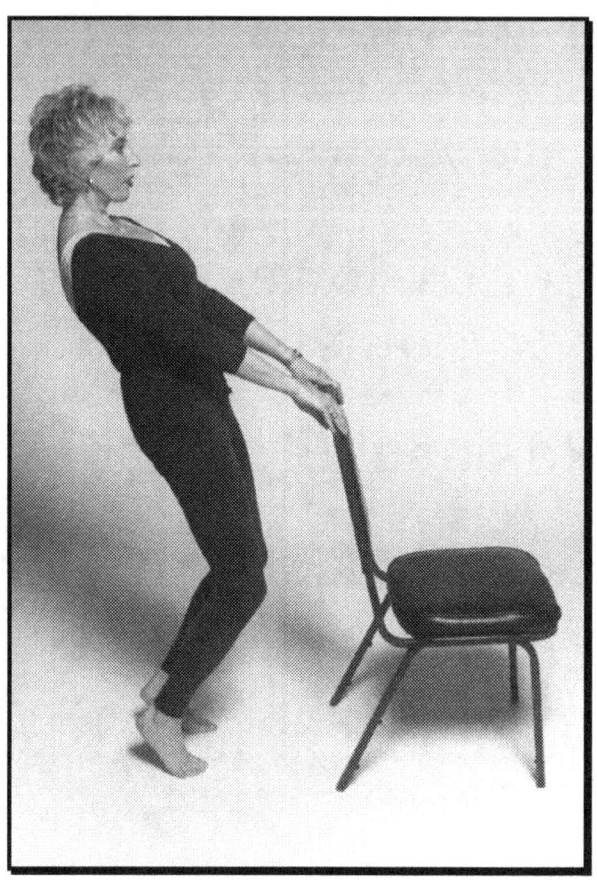

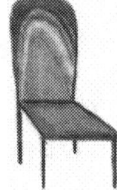  Stand tall behind chair, shoulders down, chest up. Place both hands on the chair back for support.

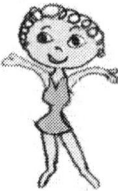 Slowly lean back rocking onto toes.

Return to a relaxed standing position.

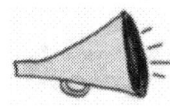 Repeat with balance and ease.

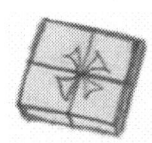 Totally terrific!

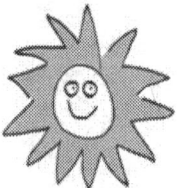

"I center myself in all that is good."

Look Behind

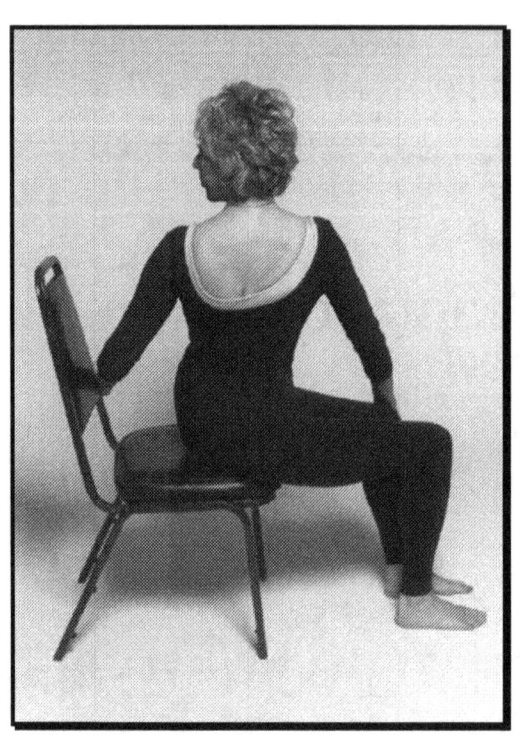 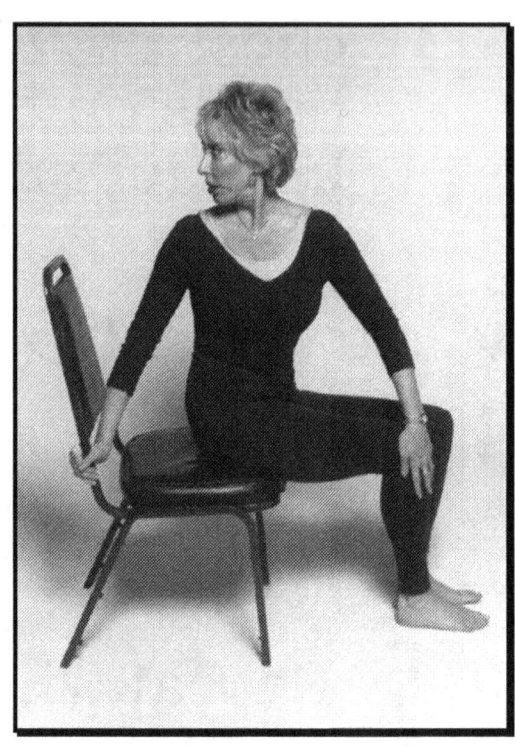

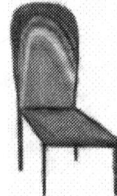  Sit tall in chair,
shoulders down,
chest up,
feet pointed forward.

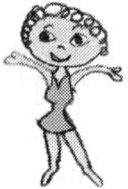 Place one hand on opposite
thigh and press as you gently
twist to look over back
shoulder.

You may want to lightly hold
onto the chair with the free
hand as you twist.

Return to a forward seated
position.

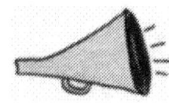 Repeat on other side.

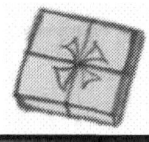 I'm proud of you!

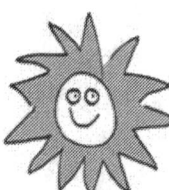

*"I look for the good
in every situation."*

Drop the Knee Look Behind

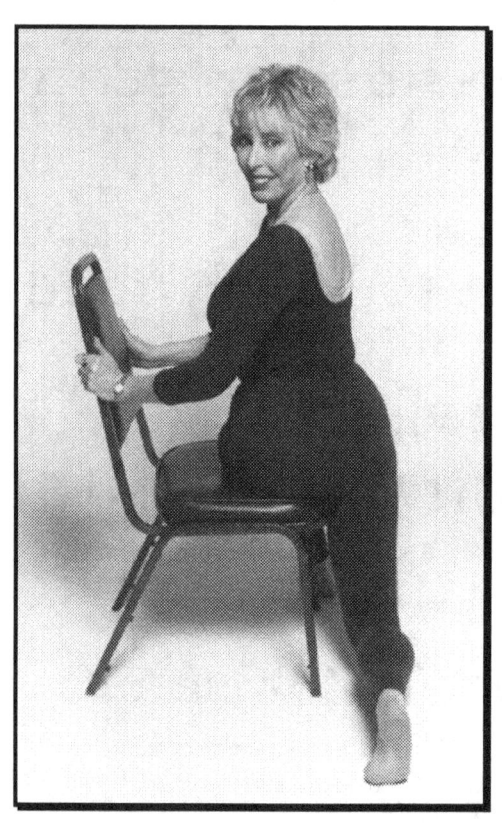 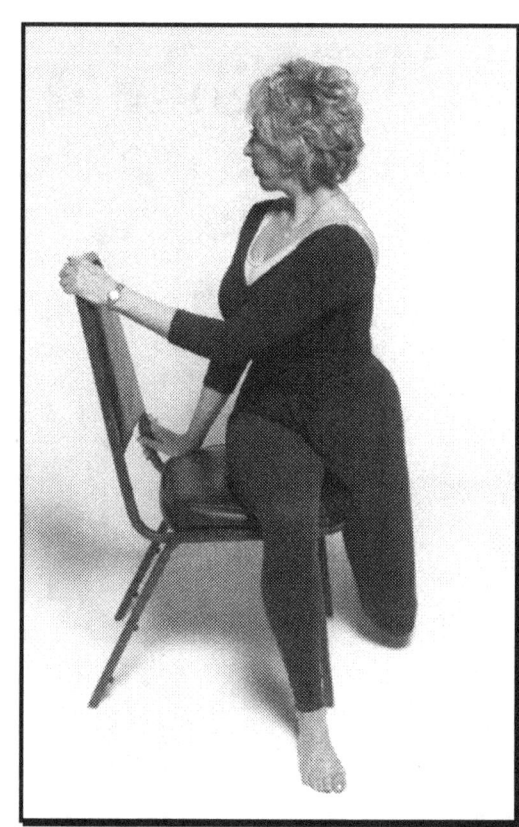

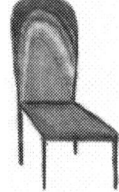  Sit tall on chair edge, shoulders down, chest up. Drop one knee to the floor.

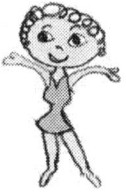 Gently twist looking behind and over the shoulder, dropping the knee and turning.

Hold the chair for support.

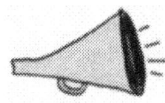 Repeat on other side.

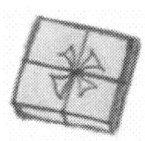 Stretch for success and smile!

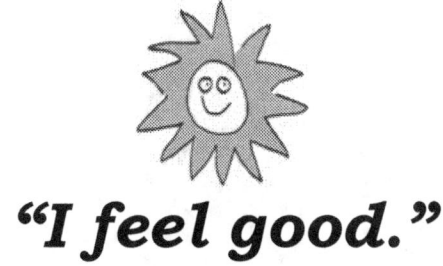

"I feel good."

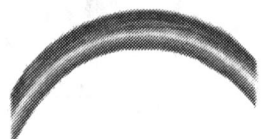

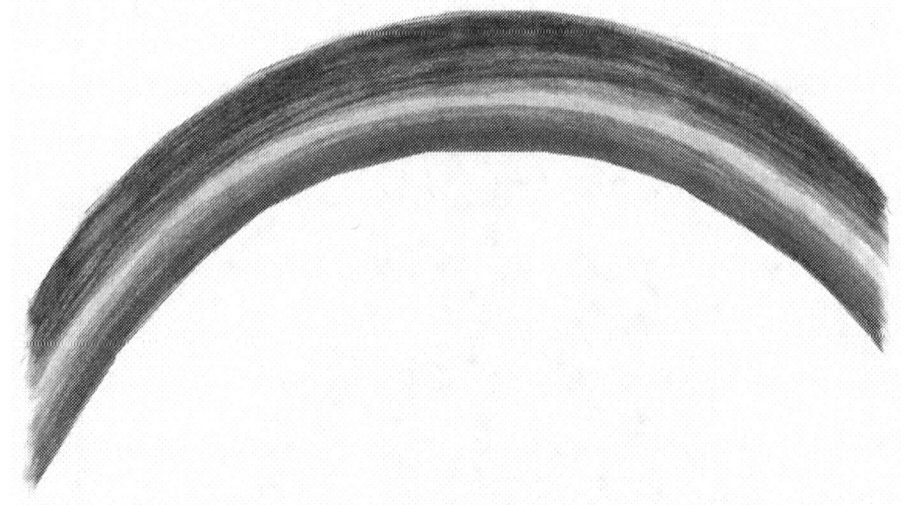

Legs &
Lower Body

Knees Out

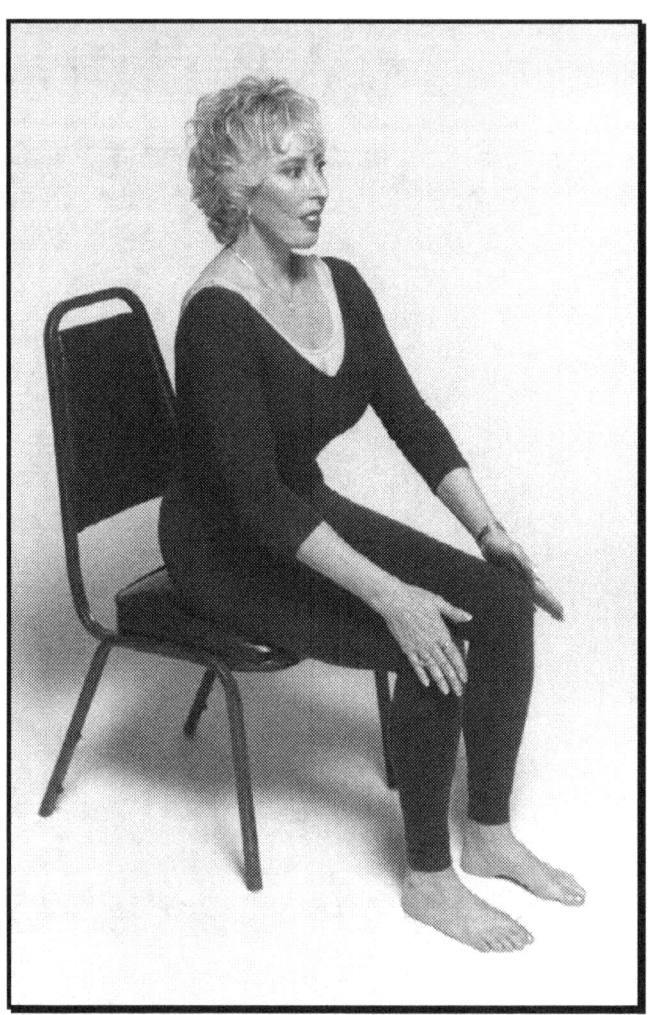

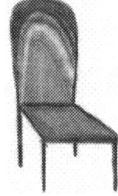 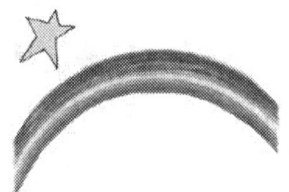 Sit tall in chair, shoulders down, chest up.

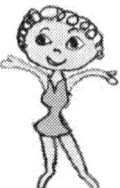 Hold the outer sides of knees.

Press legs outward.

Provide resistance with hands.

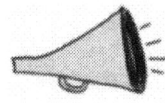 Repeat with glee.

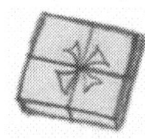 Press on!

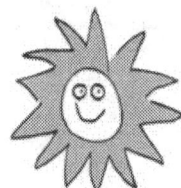

"I am powerful, peaceful and poised."

Knees In

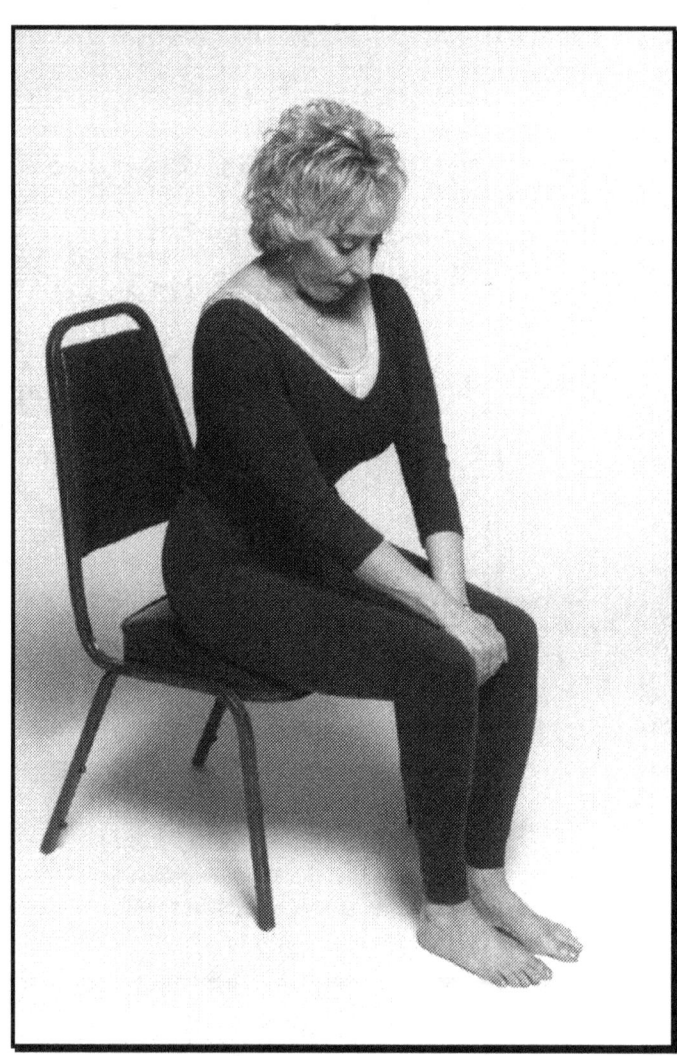

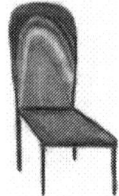 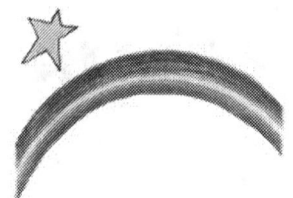 Sit tall in chair, shoulders down, chest up, feet together flat on the floor.
Belly in.

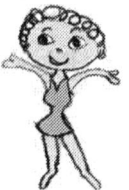 Place fists between knees.

Squeeze legs together.

Release.

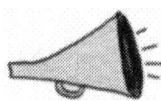 Repeat happily.

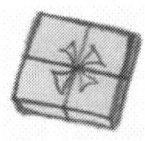 Way to go!

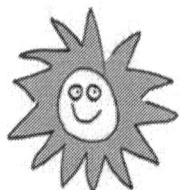

"I release and let go."

Firm Thigh

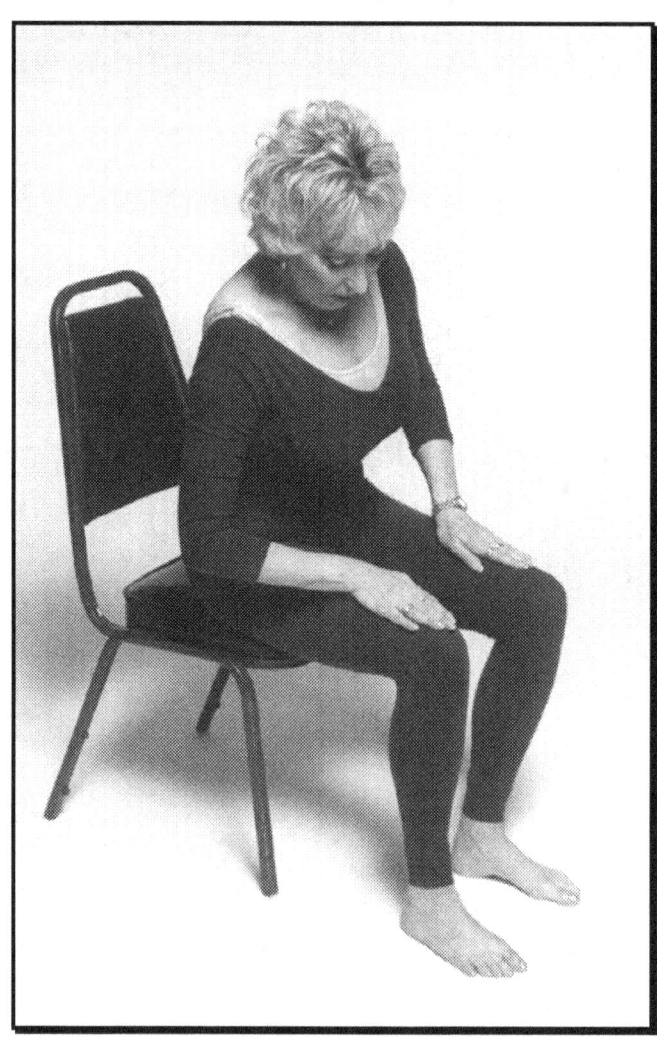

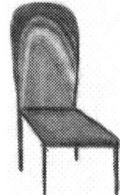 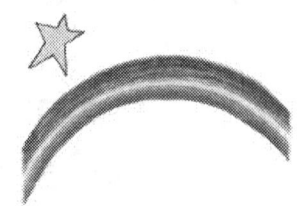 Sit tall in chair, shoulders down, chest up, with feet hip-width apart.

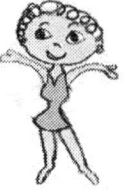 Gently press one foot down into floor, pressing down on thigh.

Hold and release.

Change leg.

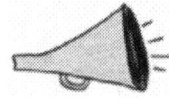 Repeat cheerfully.

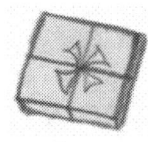 Excellent work!

"I am firmly rooted in good."

Knee Kiss

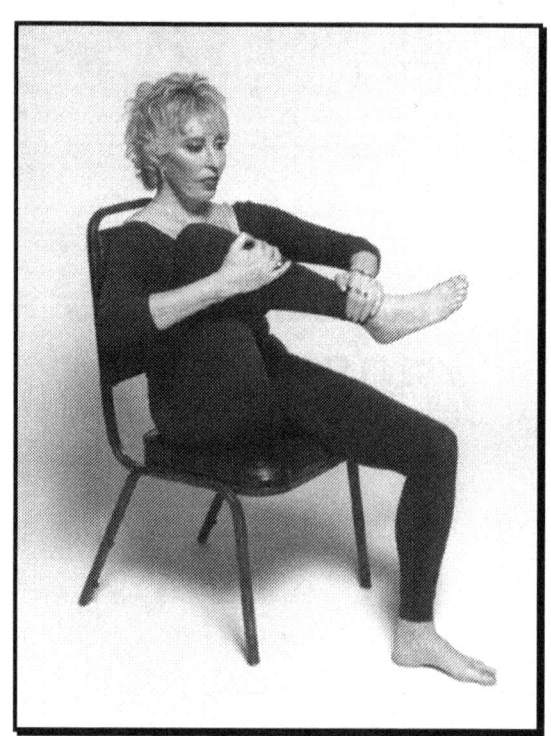
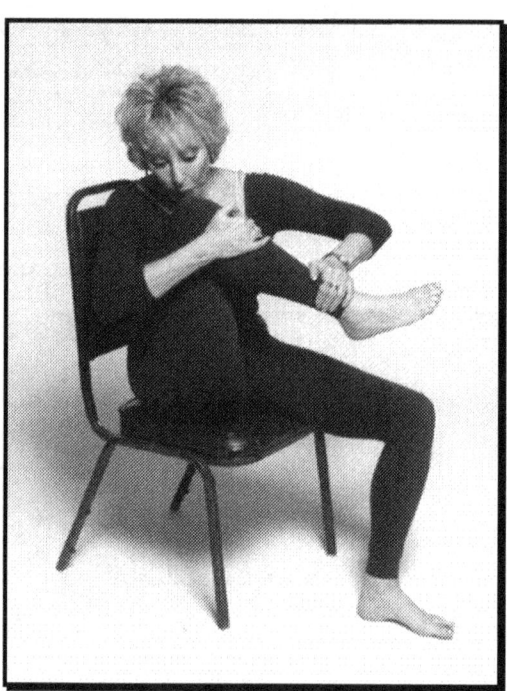
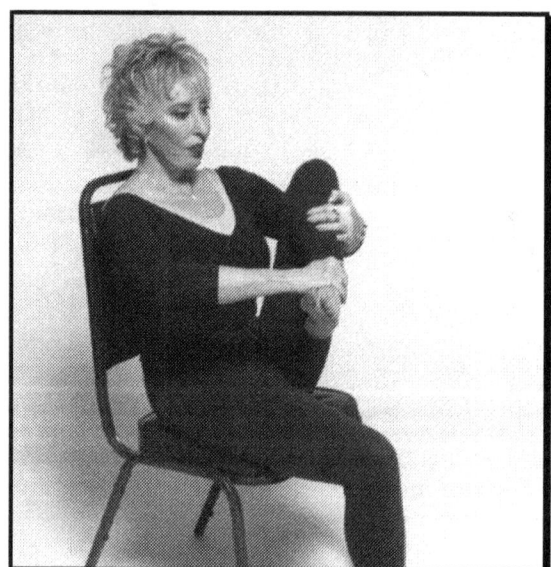
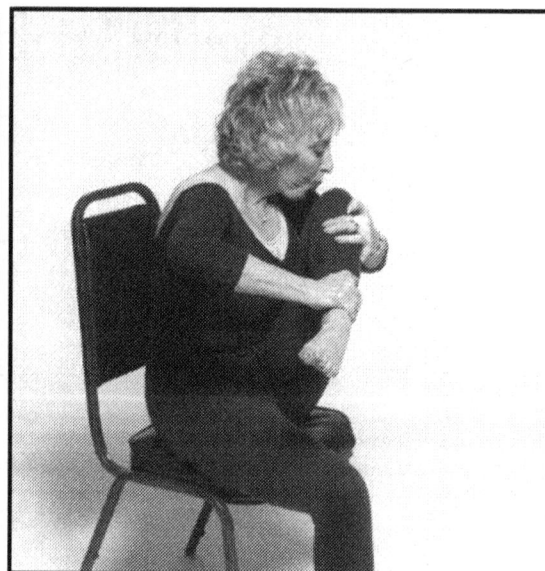

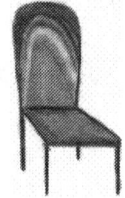  Sit tall in chair, shoulders down, chest up.

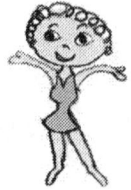 Take hold of one leg.

Lift knee gently toward chest, and if you can, give it a kiss!

Otherwise, blow it a kiss!

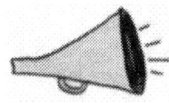 Repeat on the other side.

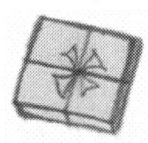 **K**eep **I**t **S**imple **S**weety.

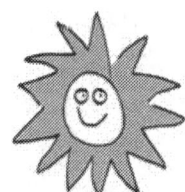

"I love myself the way I am."

Be Hip

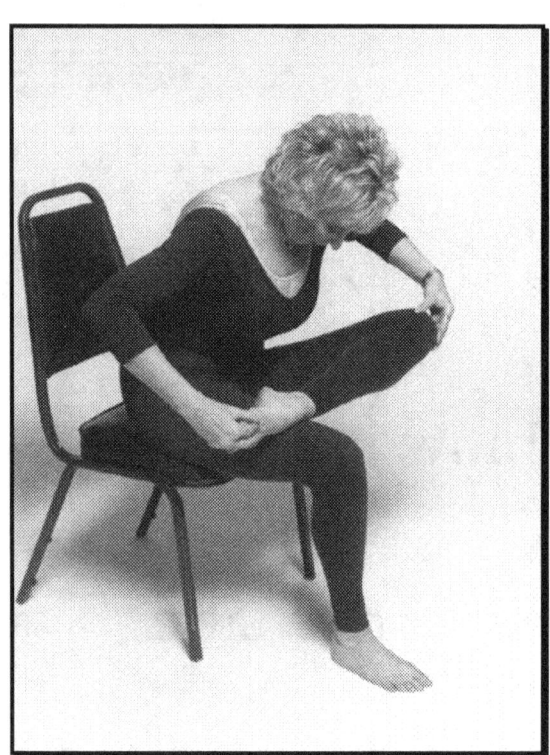 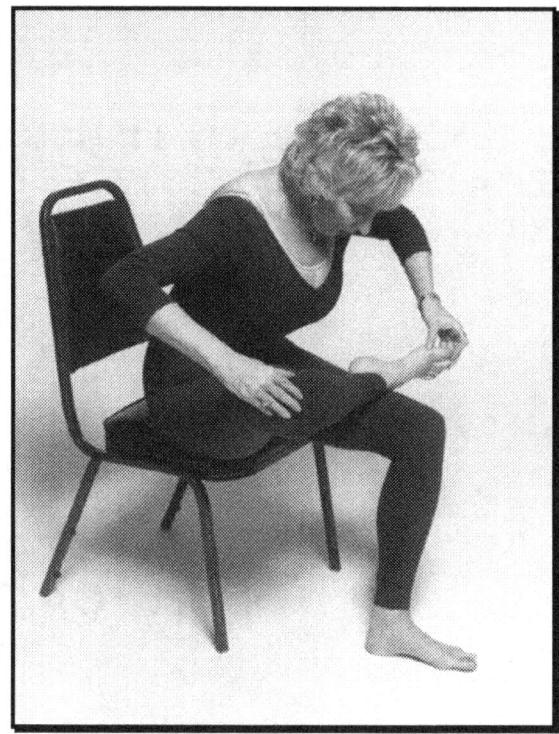

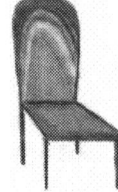  Sit tall in chair, shoulders down, chest up.

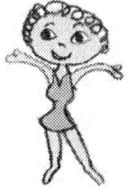 Gently cross leg.

Place ankle on thigh - inhale.

Slowly bend forward and hold - exhale.

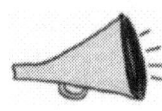 Use leg for support.

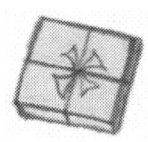 Repeat merrily on the other side.

Hip hip hooray!

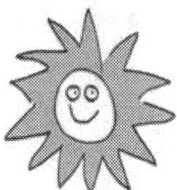

"I am flexible and capable."

Leg & Thigh Stretch

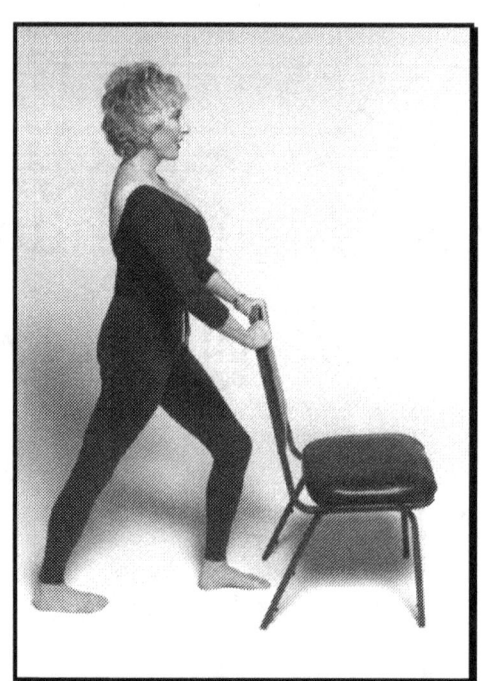 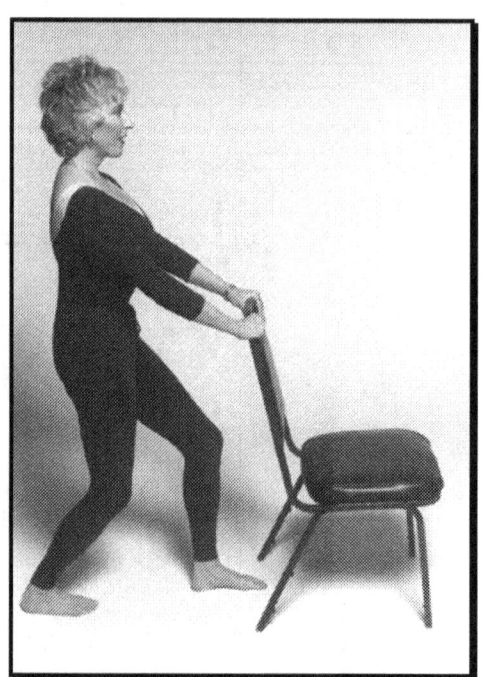

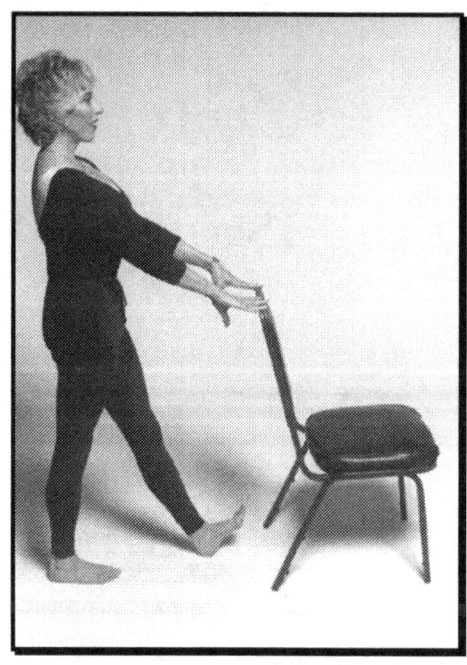

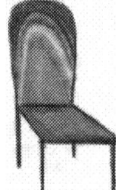

Stand tall behind chair. Place both hands on chair back. Spread feet apart, staggered one in front of the other, toes forward.

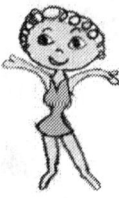

Slowly bend front knee and hold.

Now, with front knee bent, bend the back knee, keeping both heels on floor and hold.

Next, slowly shift weight to back foot and gently pull toes of the front foot up toward knee.

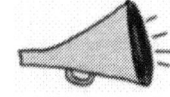

Repeat joyfully on other side.

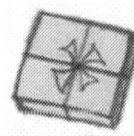

Walk the walk!

***"I move forward with ease
and comfort."***

Back Leg Lifts

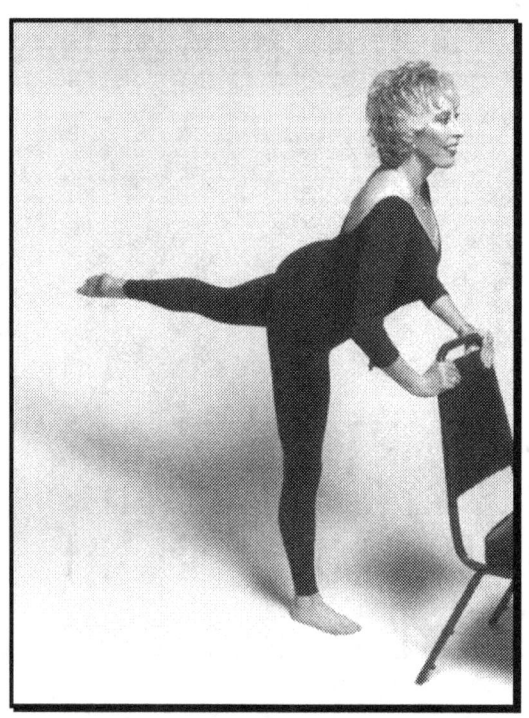 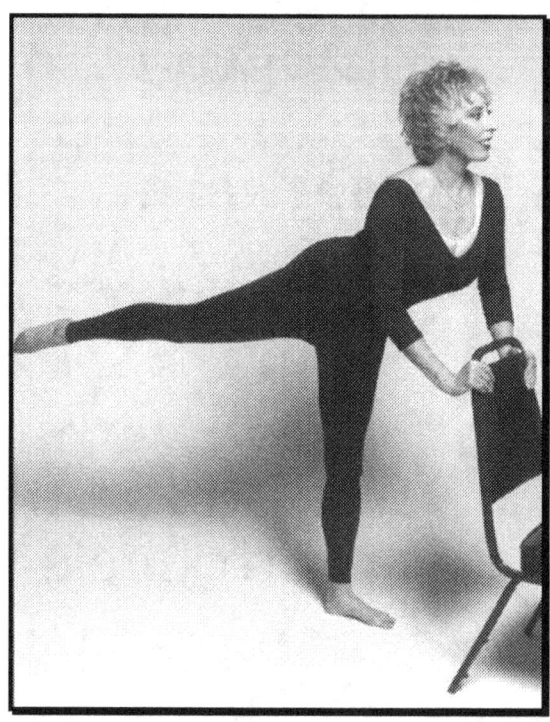

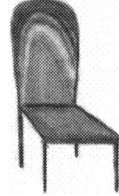 Stand tall behind chair, shoulders down, chest up. Place both hands on chair back.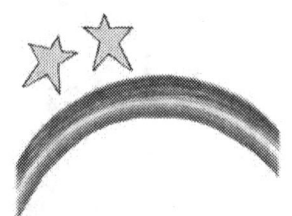

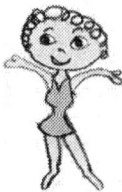 In a gentle swinging motion, raise one leg to the rear as high as is comfortable.

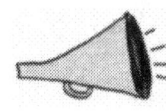 Repeat several times on each side.

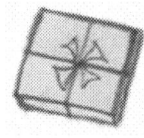 Your balance is good!

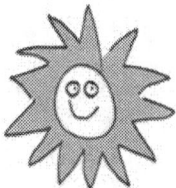

"I move with strength and power."

Side Leg Lifts

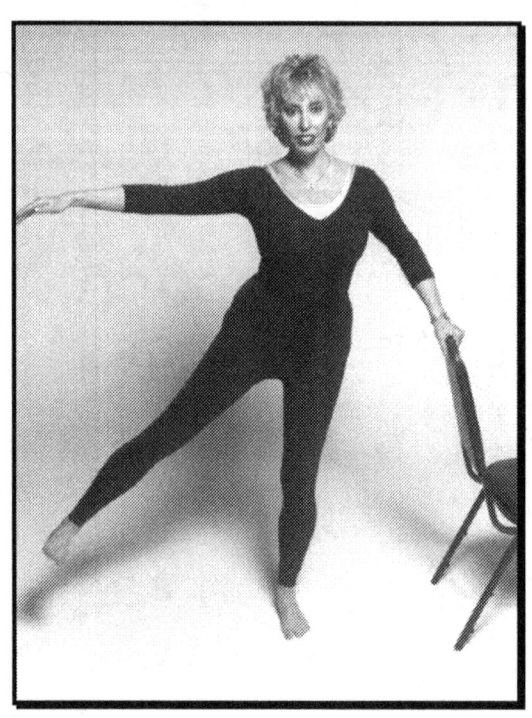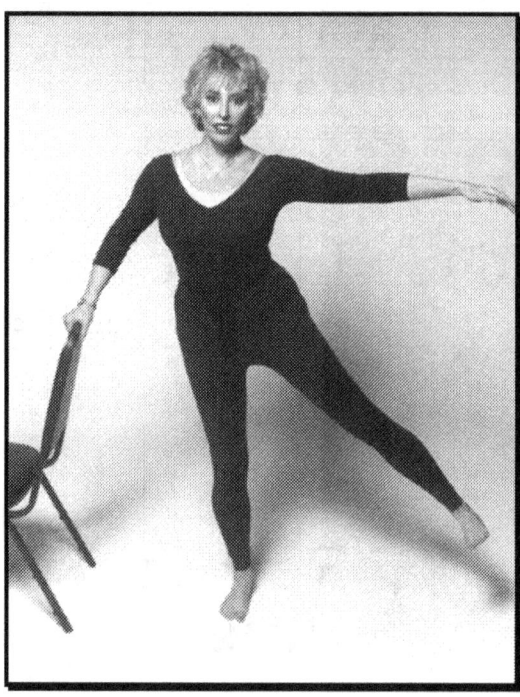

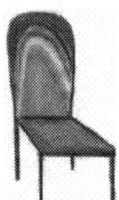
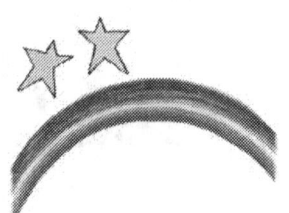

Stand tall beside chair, shoulders down, chest up. Place one hand on chair back for support.

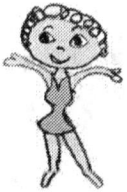

Lift other arm out to the side for balance.

Gently lift the outer leg to the side and lower it several times.

Keep it steady, knees facing forward.

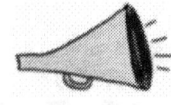

Turn and repeat on other side.

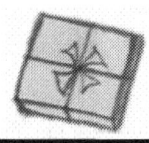

Your legs are like steel!

"In everything I do I have a leg up."

Heel Thyself

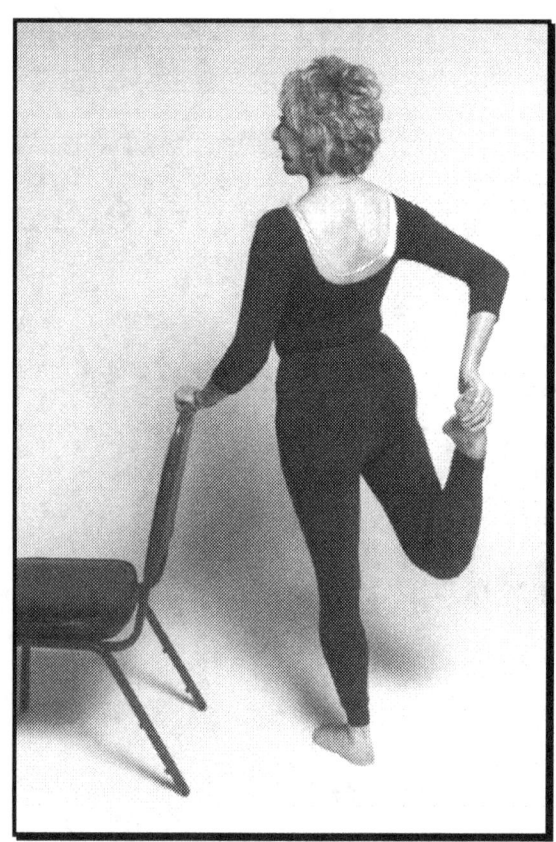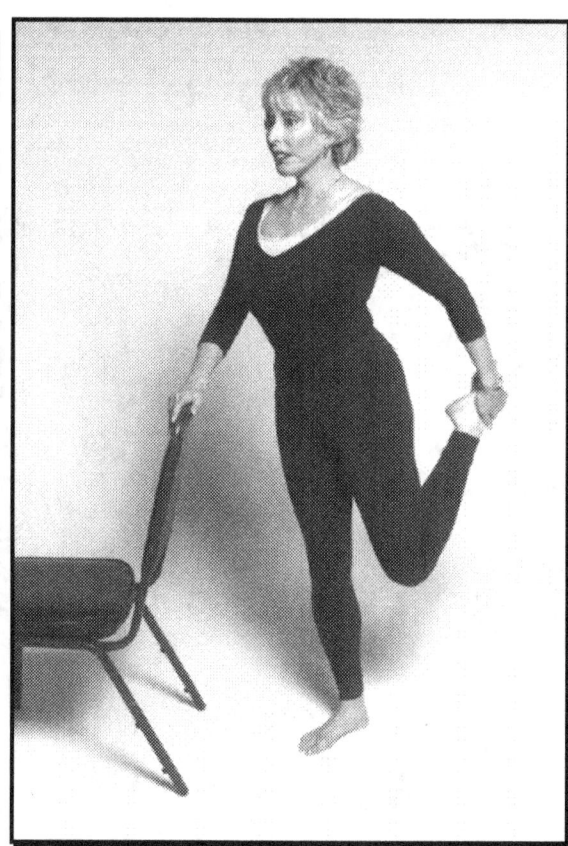

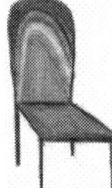  Stand tall beside chair, shoulders down, chest up. Place one hand on chair back for support.

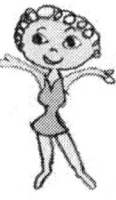 Bend outer leg back.

Hold foot.

(If you cannot hold the foot, simply stand on one foot using the chair for support.)

Relax and let go of foot.

Gently return it to floor.

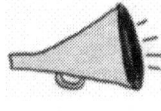 Repeat cheerfully on other side.

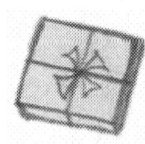 Great feat!

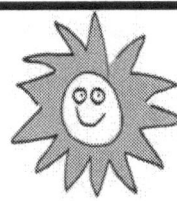

"I heal myself."

Step Up

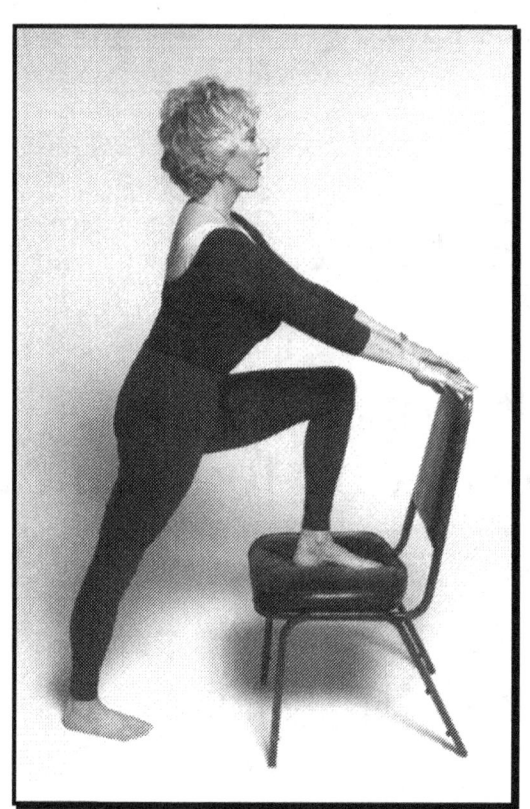 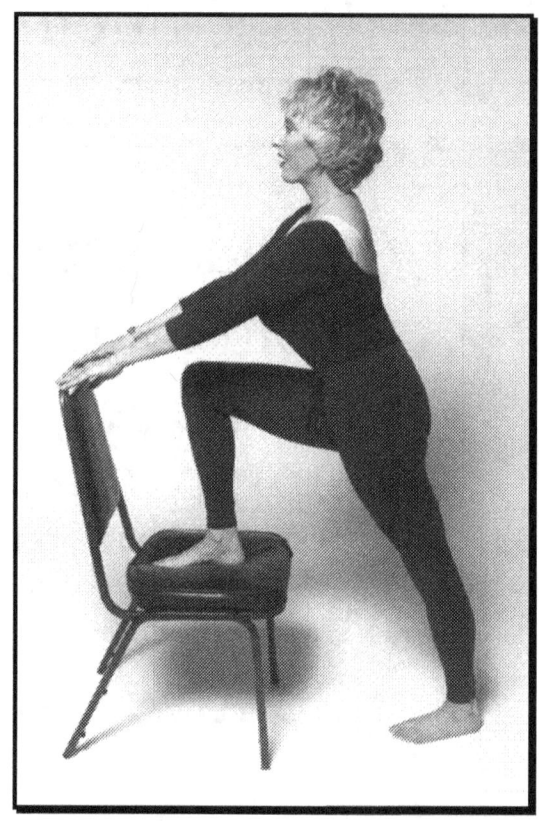

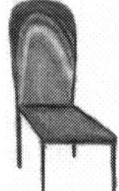 Stand tall in front of chair, shoulders down, chest up. Place both hands on chair back for support.

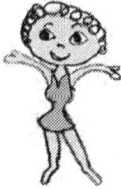 Step onto chair with one foot and stretch gently - inhale.

(If chair is too high for you, lift leg with bent knee as high as is comfortable.)

Lower leg to ground - exhale.

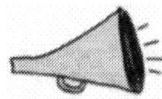 Repeat joyously with other leg.

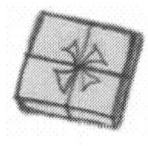 Enjoy!

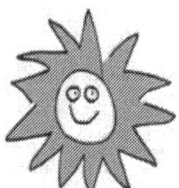

"I step up to new experiences."

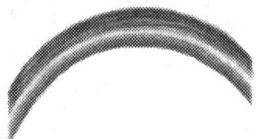

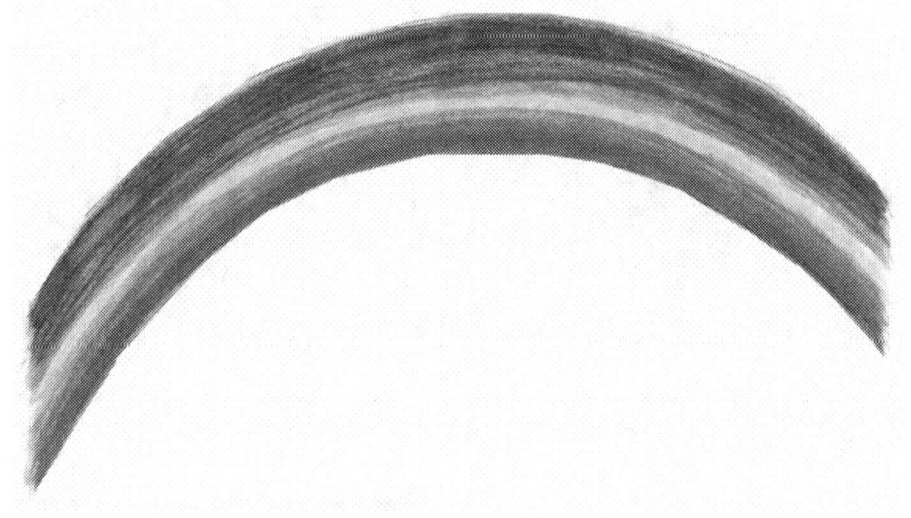

Legs,
Ankles & Feet

Toe Heel Toe

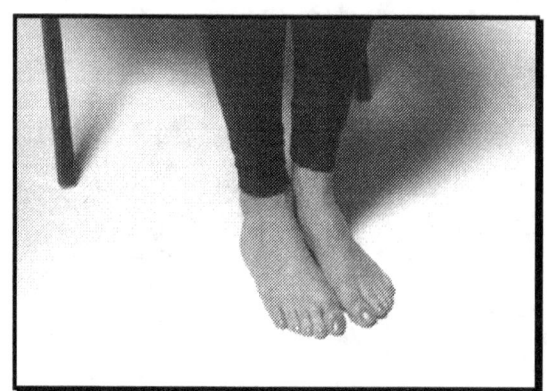
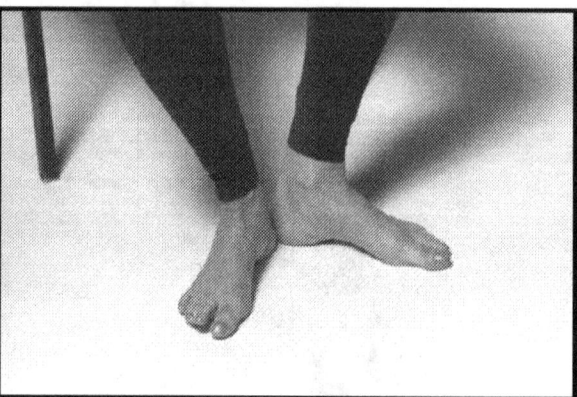

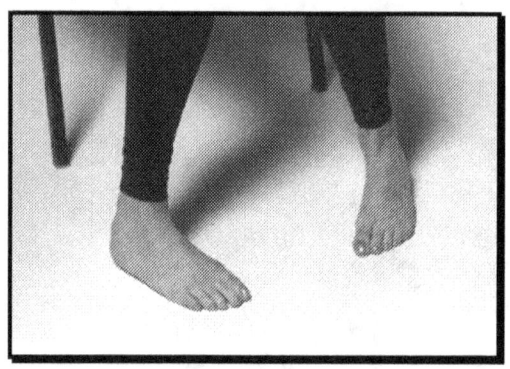
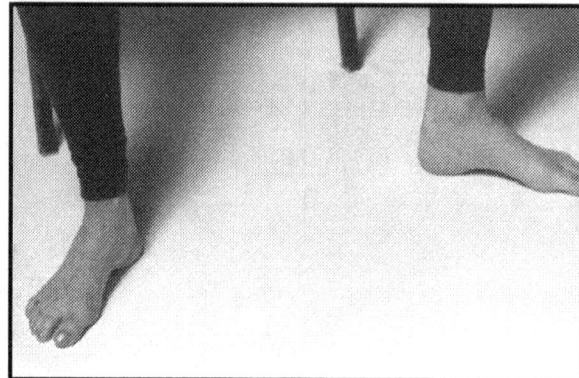

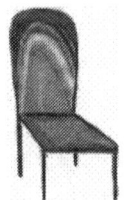  Sit tall in chair, shoulders down, chest up. Place feet together flat on floor.

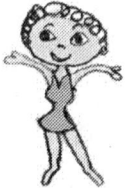 Move toes away from each other, keeping the heels together forming a "V" shape.

Next, pivot on balls of feet placing heels out - pigeon toed.

Now, move toes apart again, pivoting on heels.

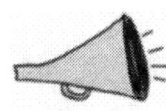 Reverse the motions to bring feet back together and repeat.

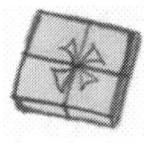 Toe heel toe. Way to go!

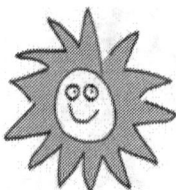

"I dance to life with happy feet and enjoy each step I take."

Toe Stretch

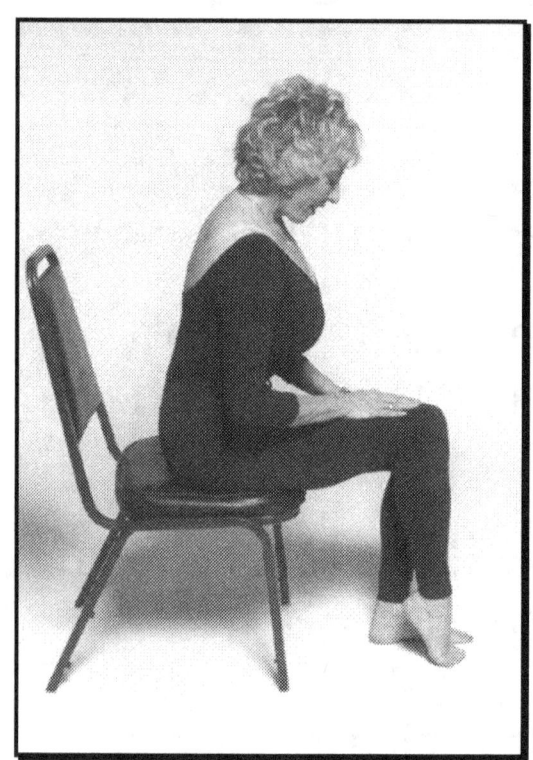

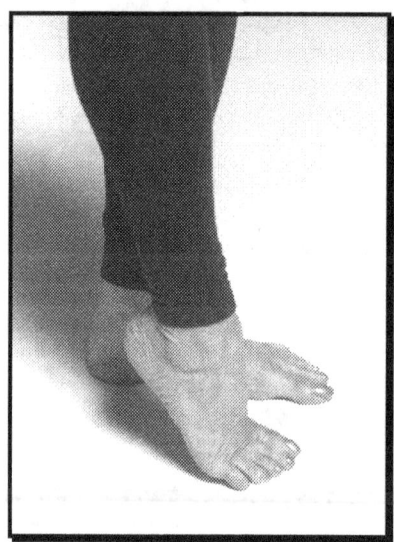

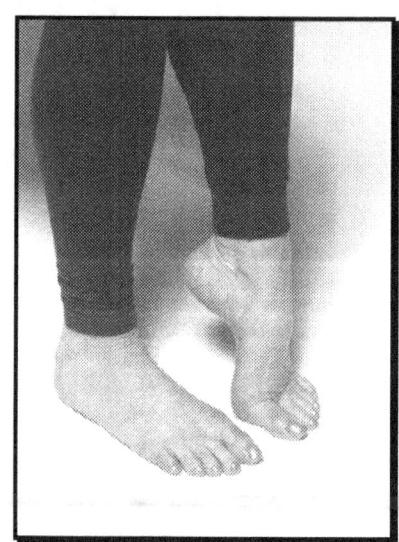

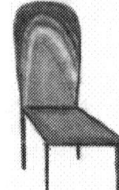 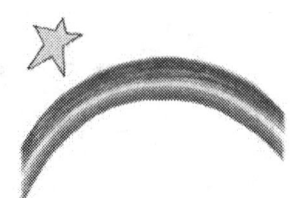 Sit tall in chair,
shoulders down,
chest up.
Place feet flat on floor.

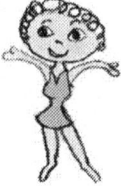 Slowly lift one heel rocking upward onto ball of foot.

Return heel to floor as you repeat the motion with opposite foot.

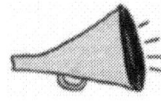 Stretch and repeat pressing toes gently into floor.

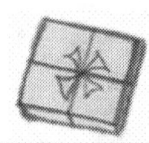 Very soleful!

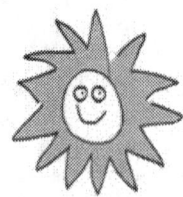

"My feet always take me in the right direction."

Feet Flip Flops

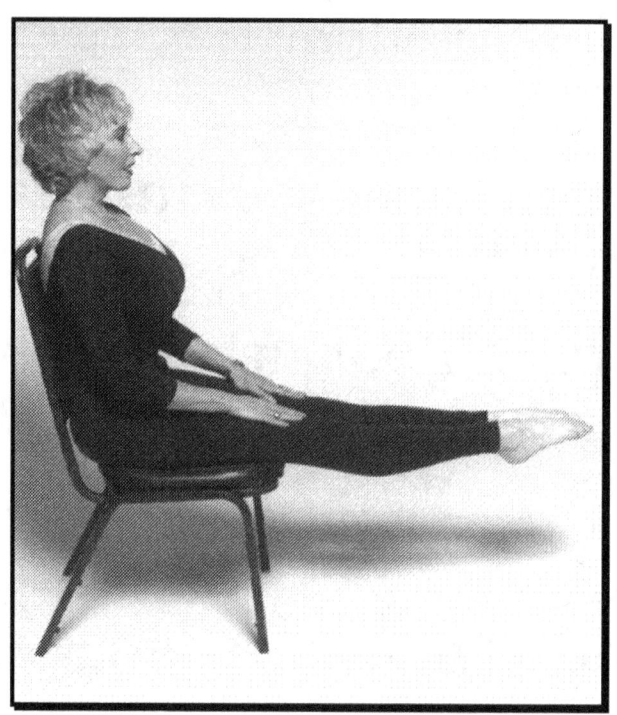

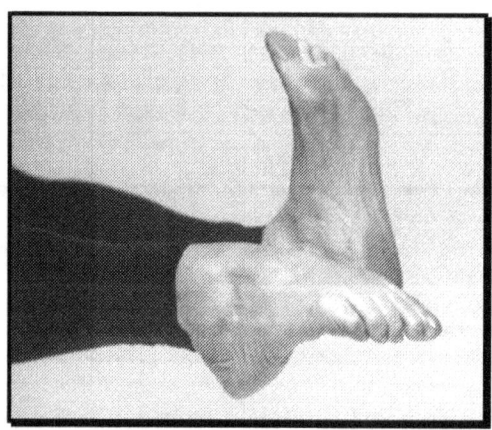
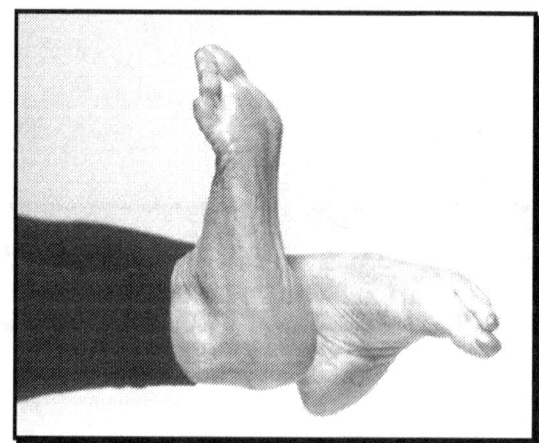

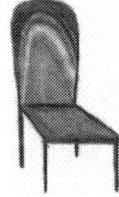 Sit in chair,
shoulders down,
chest up.

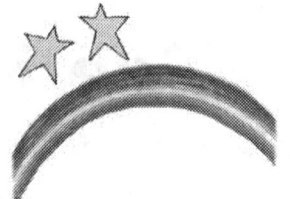

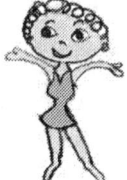 With legs extended parallel to
floor, toes pointed straight
ahead, pull toes of one foot
back, pushing heel forward.

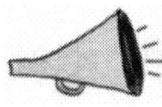 Repeat this motion with other
foot as you return first foot to
point.

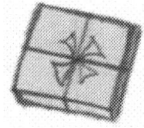 Flip flop feet.
Fabulous footwork.

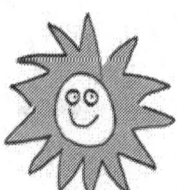

*"I dance to life
with happy feet."*

Toe Lifts

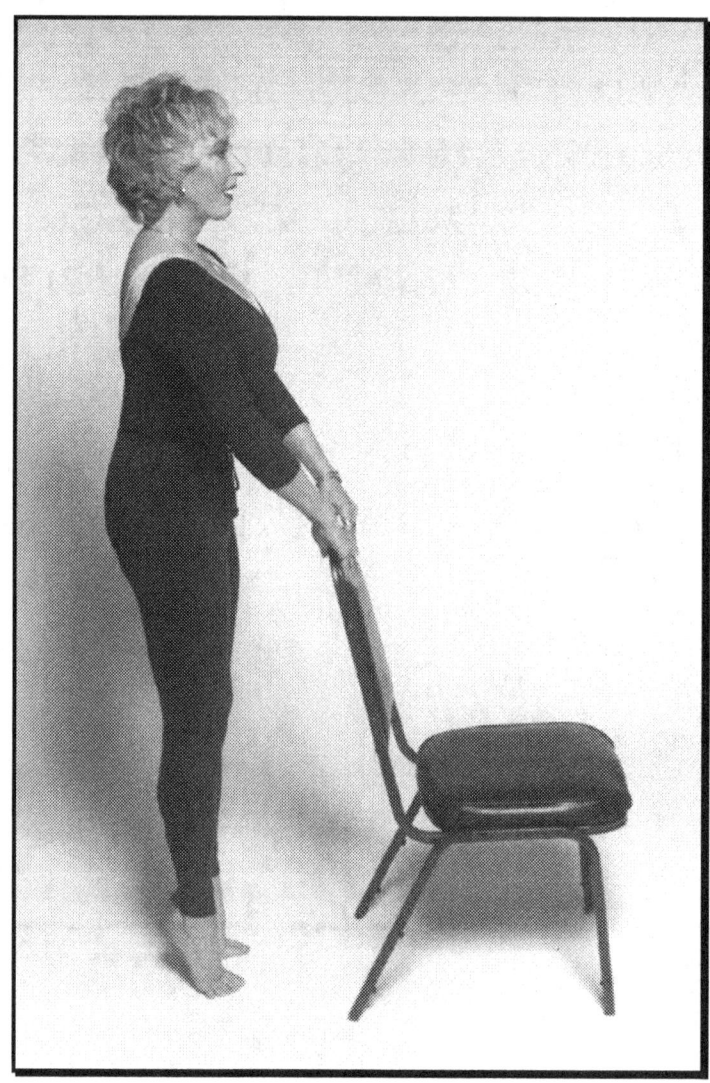

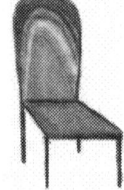  Stand tall behind chair, shoulders down, chest up. Place both hands on chair back, feet flat on ground.

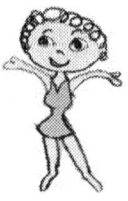 Lift heels, raising to toes.

Lower feet slowly.

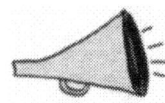 Repeat - up and down.

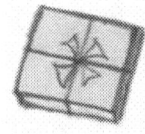 Up, up and away!

"I am inspired and uplifted."

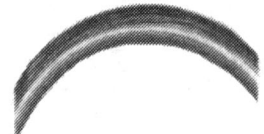

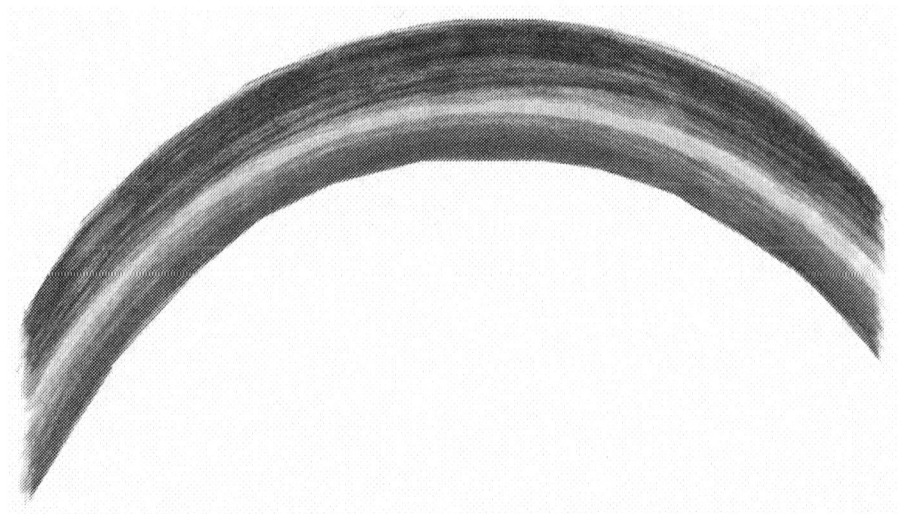

The End

...is just the beginning.

I bet you thought there would be a pot of gold waiting for you here. But as the mystics state, "it is in the journey that the seeker is found."

We must remind ourselves that the "gold" or the rainbow comes from within. This is why I couple each exercise with a positive affirmation. Each movement we make, each breath we take is holy. It is another step in the dance of life...

You have already reached your rainbow. It was there all along!

God Bless and enjoy the journey.

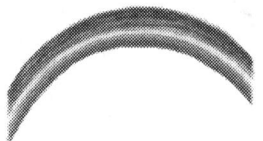

About the Author

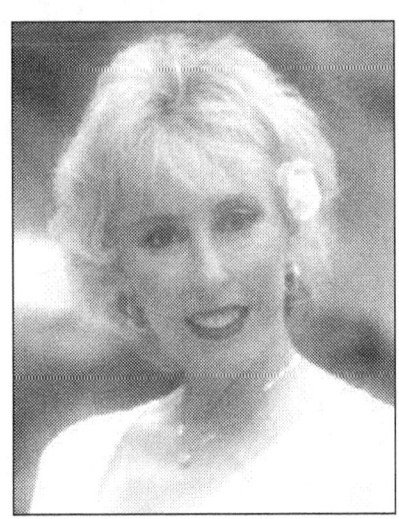

Brenda L. Rogers is a nationally acclaimed fitness consultant. She has appeared on television programs and has worked with celebrities from talk show hosts to Academy award winners.

As a personal and corporate fitness pioneer, she has designed stress reduction and exercise programs for Rockwell International, Hughes Aircraft, and Redken Laboratories. Ms. Rogers has been a staff member for hospitals and healthcare organizations. As a dance professional, lecturer, and relaxation therapist, she provides classes in movement and creative expression.

Ms. Rogers facilitates longevity courses as a certified senior wellness instructor. She is a licensed practitioner and spiritual counselor.

Ms. Rogers has two sons and currently resides in Washington State.

Order Form

Those who would like to receive information about Brenda L. Rogers' workshops, lectures, events, or products may fill out, detach, and mail the form below.

NAME:

_____

ADDRESS:

_____

PHONE:

_____

EMAIL:

_____

COMMENTS:

_____

_____

Mail to:

Brenda L. Rogers

19528 Ventura Blvd., Suite 581

Tarzana, CA 91356

www.brendarogers.com